Epilepsy Memoir: My 40-year Detour

for epilepsy awareness month and of being single and lonely. I'd love to have a girlfriend, marriage, or any of the combinations in between like living together. Love is love, that's what it amounts to and sex is sex, no matter what form the love takes. I loved my service dog and he loved me. Love; life; love and epilepsy, we all have to get our priorities right. I love you all, honestly, I do. Just remember that you are important too and I don't just mean the E people, everyone. I don't drive nor have I ever wanted to so I don't have a driver's license; transportation has always been a real bitch with me so transportation to and from the event, meals, and if necessary lodging would have to be included.

Contents

DEDICATION

This book is dedicated to the memory of Mister John Stohr, a teacher of Social Studies I had back in the late 1970s. He was forced to leave his teaching position after having two grand mal (as they were known at the time) seizures in public in a classroom. He became regional delivery manager for a major newspaper located in the Twin Cities, in Minnesota; he died tragically in a fiery seizure-related auto accident. Unfortunately, John chose to drive even though his seizures were uncontrolled. This occurred in 1980, pre- the ADA (Americans Disability Act) that would have protected his right to hold that teaching position. The short of it was that he was fired because he had Epilepsy. I got the kind permission of his mother—Angelina Stohr to dedicate the book to him. At the time I contacted her, Angelina was 93-years-old and was broken up over the fact that two of her sons had died before her; John was one of those sons. Anyway, I hope she is still living when this book is published and I am able to get a copy to her. However, that was over a decade ago, and chances are she didn't live to be over 100. Wherever you rest now Angelina, thank you for your kindness.

INTRODUCTION

I'm going to keep this simple; I'm going to practice my honesty—even if it hurts, and some memories, particularly alcohol and what happened in a classroom are painful. I was told when I started this particular project that it would be a healing experience for me, and that's true.

I had three women of varying ages I befriended on the Epilepsy Foundation site, one in her 20s, one in her 30s, and one in her 50s - read through the final draft of my memoir manuscript and all gave thumbs up positive reviews. One shared opinion was that it was a lot of information in a small package or in keeping with the concept, a compact car. Many thanks go out to those three E ladies for taking time out of their busy schedules.

Life Motto for a Single Man trying his damned best to make a living with his writing, coping…

Love is love, no matter whom, or what or when, love is love. Coping means loving yourself, to mentally touch yourself and bring joy to your life, bring happiness to yourself and not feel guilty about being happy and hope others are as happy as you are in a mental and physical way…there are many types of happiness to be experienced. Give others a hand up but don't forget yourself as you do, never forget that you are important too. Please be as sexual as you want or feel you want to be. I am extremely open-minded about sexuality and not meaning by any means that I'm hetero, am homo, am asexual, or a term I've come up with, uni-sexual that covers the solo-sex pioneers.

I'm what I call a Christian realist meaning that I know that there's a hell of a lot that can be done medically than with religiosity. To give you an idea how off the wall these Bible-thumpers can get, last Sunday I went down to my home away from home for Arnie Palmer and steak and eggs, my usual religious day repast. I was just sitting there by myself bothering no one like a good little 54-year-old boy and a woman who by all previous appearances began thumping that holy book and began scratching in her purse for her magic wand crucifix. Like I said, I was bothering no one when this woman who I'll call Bertha "big-butt" Johnson said, "You know Donald, what have you been up to," it always starts out as a bad day when somebody uses your full name. There had been a Facebook post by someone I'll call Vicky the open-legged sexual vixen. Vicky has more of an appearance of slimy quick dry cement or lutefisk white sauce or thick and lumpy semen—I do know what that stuff looks like from firsthand experience—that is I could see it was slimy and lumpy. I'd had a long seizure, maybe 45 minutes or maybe 2 hours on Thursday, this was a Sunday as I'd returned from my parents for our weekend free food—my brother and I almost always go up there on the weekends—I posted that I thought the reason that I had the seizure was heat, I overheat and I seize. Vicky went religious on me, "We are powerless over them bullcrap yada yada bullcrap... we should all turn our lives over to God to heal us of our affliction." I'm not atheist, not agnostic, but that is a load of frozen horse apples. She and I had a one sided disagreement in which I told why I mentioned religion and God as little as possible in this book, I wanted it universal, for the Islamic and Buddhists and Jews, the Christians and atheists and agnostic, that epilepsy is race color-blind and that epilepsy didn't care how much pigment was in your skin, whether you were thin or fat, large breasted or small, 6-years-old or 96. Did you know that the highest prevalence for epilepsy was age 2 or younger or age 75 and older. I wrote it for cops and clergy, docs and GPs, shrinks and therapists, Moms and Dads and brother, sister, and Aunt or Uncle. Then there are friends. When my friend Walt and I had a dual author signing I sold 11 books mostly to friends of my parents, I think Walt sold 3. For the RP of Detour that was the first name of this memoir. Miller, you did it again, I went off on a tangent. Vicky and I differed in our religious points of view. So that Sunday, I tell Bertha about the post and that I went off on Vicky who was busy spouting religious clap-trap. I said, "Epilepsy is not supernatural, E people are not demonically possessed," "Oh, yes they are," I must really be a slow learner, now I've only had epilepsy for 43 years but epilepsy is supernatural, "Oh, yes, it is and here's a religious tract that will educate your mind right." The name of the religious tract she dug out of her purse was, and I really got a kick out of the title, a kick in the testicles that is, GROUP PRAYER CIRCLE, PRAY FOR MIRACLE CURES, that's bunk with a capital B. I know religious stuff, have read the Bible from Genesis to Revelations, been baptized, confirmed Lutheran, became a member of Zion Lutheran and maybe the miracle cures thing works for paralysis and blindness, in the Bible I think it says, and JC Superstar made the lame to walk and the blind to see. That same

JC gave the E people a bum rap, convulsing man, demonical-ly possessed, my name is Legion as my numbers are 1000 demons (it's something like that), demons take a hike, a herd of pigs go mad and jump over the edge of a cliff, bloody mess on the hillside. Back to Bertha, as she and Randolph were leaving I waited until they were at the door, when Bertha turned around probably to lay down more religious smack on me and call me a blasphemous hypocrite I threw the single fingered salute in her direction, the bird, the American Eagle. I caught a flash of light and it might have been a trick of the light but I think that Randy winked at me and thought, 'oh no, not again.' Now if you're a believer and prayer works for you, bully and yeah for you. I'm a Christian realist. Now, back to the book, about the lumpy semen, even at my advanced age, I've qualified for an AARP membership for 4 years now. I've written a query letter to AARP, the magazine and hope to write a series of epilepsy Zen arti-cles—my latest memoir is Holistic Zen & the NASCAR epilepsy ninja: You can overcome epilepsy disability abuse & Myths about epilepsy broken you should check it out—I'm going to include a copy of the book with the query letter so they could check it out. It is an epilepsy memoir but no more like a biography than a bull is to a chicken (city boy, I have no idea about farm stuff), I'm not sure what a cultivator is or what exactly it is that you do with it. I did it again, lumpy, slimy semen, even at the age of 54 I occasional have a nocturnal emission or blow my load off into the sheets. That takes a lot of detergent to get out if it gets out at all. In that letter to AARP, I've done 3 or 4 drafts I mentioned senior and disability masturbation. That particular topic made me a little uncomfortable as people could have thought I masturbated; after all I am one of the disabled. I mentioned orgasm anesthesia also. I believe I mention this book in the bibliography in back; it was a Writer's Digest Book Club Book of the Month Selection titled Sex for One: the Joy of Self-loving and Betty Dodson also known as the mother of masturbation give a pretty graphic description of that topic and bisexuality, homosexuality, also oral sex. I remember that I kept sex out of the book entirely but we are sexual beings with sexual needs that need to be fulfilled, I don't get what the big deal is about masturbating—I better rephrase that I know what gets big and hard—but I really don't get what the big deal is about the activity or why you need to. There is a lot of sex talk in my Epilepsy Zen book, virgin of 26 meets virgin of 23, things get a little sweaty and experiment and we had mutual love each other; that is from my point of view. Cherry Stovington, as hot in temperament as she was hot in sexual desires, she was very familiar with that activity. She had deep auburn hair, cornflower blue eyes, black pubic hair that was cushiony like an Afro. Sometimes we'd check which way the pubic hair was growing on each other. It was called one of the bases, first, maybe second and we never rounded the base path for a home run as we were both virgins when we split and never went as far as intercourse. And what is the big deal about virginity? In 2013 I went off of Dilantin and onto Banzel while at United hospital, unit 4900, Intensive Monitoring Suites. I remember getting an erection—a hard-on—when in the same room as a Neuro-psych tech who was a real knockout. If she saw I was engorged and a little uncomfortable, chafing and pressure she was kind of nice not to say anything about although being that I was 49 I wouldn't have minded a little pressure relief. One nurse just for the sake of a name was Wendy, a redhead, beautiful girl, beautiful green eyes, she said she came from Stillwater, Minnesota, the town I grew up in. I remembered another Wendy, a redhead, beautiful girl, beautiful green eyes and I wondered if it was the same person, in life you never know. Miller, you've gone off on a tangent. We proceeded to have a sexual discussion, she said that I should be celibate or masturbate (that kind of rhymes) because of the frogs in the pond. She explained that she was really into herbal cigarettes and I could almost swear she'd been smoking some pot beforehand. It got a bit embarrassing when she explained what intercourse was and sodomy—it turned out that was one of her favorites—oral sex, something called Italian style, doggy style and then she gave the reason I should do any of them with a female or a male. I'm really open-minded but still at the age of 54 I'm a virgin on both sides. Then she explained about the frogs in the pond. It turns out that there was a pond in back of a pharmaceutical company where frogs were breeding. It was also where they disposed of pills that had expired. All sorts of birth defects occurred—according to her, of course she probably was high at the time, why else the frank discussion of sex—she said again to be celibate or masturbate (that really does rhyme) and I've been celibate from age 15 on. In Victorian times—and this has to be one of the most lame epilepsy myths—they thought that epilepsy was caused by excessive masturbation. Just what quota amount was excessive. It also seems to imply that all Victorians masturbated from the Pope to the queen of England and Prussia and Sweden to monks and bishop and cardinals and boys and girls. Everybody, if so it must really have reeked like dead fish. So I agreed, no sex, I hadn't been Cherry's lover in 22 years so it wasn't likely to happen anyway. This is mentioned in the new book but it is one of the most bizarre conversations I've ever had, I think the year was 2008 and I get a call from Cherry, I have no idea where she got my number, it's in the book but probably the Internet. She was always one for her booze and I'm fairly certain she was loaded at the time. "Don, last week my mother was back from Alabama and staying at my apartment, she broke into tears, but I wasn't going to listen to a load of bullcrap." she caught me doing that thing the church wouldn't approve of but I'm not going to stop because it feels too damn good." Now things started to add up, her failure to climax and her intimate touching of her hood and clitoris and moaning. She asked if I'd give her a hand at what she was doing. I was always an obliging lover before we split for good in 1991. I was always willing to help out. Like I said a damn bizarre conversation I call the masturbation conversation. I could tell she was naked—even after 20 years I was a little psychic—and she assumed I was also. I was because the AC in my apartment wasn't working and it had to have been in the 90s, plus I'd been epilepsy Zen meditating, I believe nudity brings us in touch with the higher astral consciousness. She said she knew I was whacking off or beating off or choking the chicken or flogging the log (just a few of the names for male masturbation) and that I probably blew my load all over my chest just like old times sake. "I know you're remembering me because I'm remembering you as she was humping her hand. Like I said, a really bizarre conversation, why don't you pick up my Epilepsy Zen book at the following website to get to full story of probably the most bizarre conversation I had with a therapist in the Zen of Mental Health and Hugging. Remember to check out the latest memoir at www.amazon.com/author/millerdon and hope to have an audio-book on Amazon, on iTunes, and on Audible like I have my first memoir Detour: a 40-year epilepsy memoir, it was released 5-22-15. Maybe it was 2016. One writer's group member said it—a reference to the religious zealot encounter—should go off like water off a duck's back, when I hear that all I can picture is ostriches with their heads stuck in the sand. What you see then is a lot of ugly bird butt.

Controversial myths about epilepsy:

1. People who have epilepsy are demonically possessed.

2. Epilepsy is supernatural.

3.   A Social Worker once told me that I went to Special Ed and couldn't possibly have a high-school diploma because "People with epilepsy are stupider than other people," I believe she meant less intelligent than but hey, what would a professional writer with three books to his credit who formats, proofreads, and edits his own work know about grammar, syntax, pronouns, prepositions, articles, formats his own and others paperbacks and e-book, no, nothing I guess because according to her I'm stupider than everyone else.

4.   E people who practice full disclosure need to be holistically adjusted and given a caffeine enema.

5.   It was never illegal for an E-person to get married. (For a long time it was illegal for E-people to get married, the next two are sort of connected to that.)

6.   Epilepsy people can't fall in love (want to bet, I fell in love with another E person, Cherry Firestone, as hot in temperament as in sexual desires or at least infatuation at the time.)

7.   It was never illegal for E-women to get pregnant; at one time children of E parents were illegal.

8.   This one doesn't make a hell of a lot of sense to me, in Victorian times they thought that epilepsy was caused by excessive masturbation, oh, yeah, that makes sense, and just what in the heck is this excessive stuff, does this mean that all Victorians masturbated. I found this golden tidbit of wisdom on the Epilepsy Foundation site.

9.   Famous people never ever get epilepsy. Want to bet, Margaux Hemingway, Richard Burton, Hugo Weaving, Florence Griffith—Flo-Jo—Joyner nicknamed by sports media as the fastest woman in the world for her gold-medal track abilities. Ms. Joyner died in 1998 when she suffocated to death in a nocturnal—nighttime—seizure. And the list goes on, Lindsey Buckingham of Fleetwood Mac, the singer composer musician Prince, Neil Young (singer and composer), Bud Abbott of the Abbott & Costello comedy team, if you look at any of their slapstick routines it is Lou Costello that does the falls and face-plants because they didn't want Abbott striking his head and going into a seizure. Nope, nobody famous there. What about Coach Jerry Kill of the Minnesota Golden Gophers, Julius Caesar, Theodore Roosevelt, Leonardo DaVinci, Michelangelo? I think Hannibal and Alexander the great but don't quote me on the last two. Supposedly the son of Genghis Khan had epilepsy. Marco Polo was supposed to have performed first aid on him, the Khan was deeply ashamed that his son was seen in one of his attacks. Khan is supposed to have his own son assassinated just because he had the mystery disease and was seen in a seizure. I don't know if the Marco Polo part was nothing more than a fairytale and there is no way of verifying that his son had epilepsy. Coach Kill took early retirement due to his uncontrolled epilepsy and other health problems. Hugo Weaving—he is an actor that played the head bad guy in the movie Matrix and Elrond in the Tolkien movies—his epilepsy has been controlled for either 18 or 20 years. I'd like to

take him out to a cafe and pick his mind over a couple cups of de-café coffee. Being an actor I'm sure he's in contact with producers on a constant basis and that this and my previous memoirs would be great documentary material. Hugo would make a great my first neurologist that I fictionalized as Regent Jacksonian. Possibly Wil Wheaton for me, Phoebe Cates or Teal Roberts if they are still acting as Seneca Summers. Patrick Stewart or Ed Harris as Jack Tate and I'll leave the casting of John Stohr, of Cecelia Jovanovich, of John Ford, and of Robert Gumnit open. I have no idea for the blond-haired neon turquoise-eyed Psych tech or for the anonymous nurse who got a surprise and said oh, my goodness. The female touch, at least I don't think I ejaculated. Maybe Clare Danes. That's just some hypothetical casting.

10.   E people were divine, the root word of epilepsy is epilambanein that means touched or seized by God, that does not mean that I or any other E person is divine. Kind of connected is E people are visionaries, only in my fiction. Certain 3rd world tribes made E people witch doctors or spirit ghost men and withheld any medication so they'd have psychic visions that helped lead the tribe.

11.   E people can ingest pounds of poisonous shit medication with no ill effect; from AED my liver has the consistency of burned Yugoslavian Yak steak. Psych side effects are often worse than the physical, double vision, imbalance, unsteady gait, ED, virginity, and on and on for physical effects, psych can include depression, extreme agitation, suicidal ideations, self-harm, hearing voices. I'm not exactly sure

just what an ideation is but it sounds nasty. I'll explain how that works: anti-epilepsy-drugs are processed by the brain, the brain is home of the psyche, drugs can lead to psychiatric unpleasantness.

12. E people can have all the caffeine they want and have no effect on their seizure control, as Doc P explained it to me, there is a neurotransmitter in the brain that clamps down on seizure activity, one cup of coffee and that chemical is cut in half. That 2-liter bottle of Jolt Cola cuts it in half again, and again until your seizure threshold is lowered to the point that you begin seizing. More on seizure threshold in a few Zen chi Chapters, the Zen of Brownies at the Christmas Book Club Party, it was entirely my fault and I bear the scars on my face to remember it.

13. E people can lower their carb intake all they want with no problems, again from Doc P, "Don't you dare lower your carbs or you'd screw—maybe she said fool—with your ketosis, ketosis is something like regulating your blood sugar, ketosis is also the root word for the Ketogenic diet that is sometimes used to treat epilepsy in children.

14. Smoking weed will control your seizures, no, and again no, it is the CBD or cannabinoid oil that is used. CBD will not make you high or cause a mental disconnect from this world like smoking weed will. Smoking weed, also known as burning rope will cause apathy so a person never gets anything done. Anis Tahar, registered pharmacist was talking about how good medical marijuana worked in controlling your

seizures and insisted that I ask Doc Jovanovich. Now I have to explain a little about an appointment though I believe I mention it further on in the section that has the pleasure scale in it. When you go to an appointment and go up to the secretary you are handed two sheets of paper with questions on them. There is the psych sheet and the physical sheet. The psych sheet is pretty straightforward, have you had any stays in the hospital since the last appointment, have you been to the ER in the last three months? One lists body parts like eyes, ears, nose, throat, bowels, and any neurological problems other than epilepsy? (I believe they mean migraines or something else.) Bowels, any problems taking a shit (evacuating your bowels), any problems pissing, any diseases other than epilepsy in the past 6 months. There is one question that pertains to marijuana and recreational drugs. Do you use any recreational drugs and if so what are the names? When I asked about marijuana Doc said smoking doesn't do it so don't start, if so she'd have 5 patients seizure free. She said that it only works in 1 out of 10 people and mostly in children. Obviously in the recreation drugs types question some people listed weed or grass or reefer or roach or jake or Mary jane or one of the other nicknames for marijuana. Then we get to the psych sheet that has some very interesting questions that ask about depression, thoughts about self-harm (I imagine genital mutilation or worse). Then we get to the pleasure scale, 1/ I do not have any pleasure in life, 2/ I have a little pleasure in life, 3/ I have a moderate amount of pleasure in my life, 4/ I am always happy in my life, 5/ I have all the pleasure I need in my life. As far as I can tell they're trying to find out if you have a sex life and if you masturbate satisfactorily. I always answer a 6 honestly because I don't want to end up on some shrink's couch. I'm sorry to feel this way but I loathe the psych people save some of the techs who are really cute. There's more to that story in the future.

15.   A GP can treat a person's epilepsy as well as a specialist, a neurologist, may as well put an epileptologist (a neurologist specializing in epilepsy on the list. On one of my frequent ER visits (fortunately it has been a few years since I've taken that unpleasant ambulance ride) this particular doctor accused me of wanting to commit suicide and that he or she could take over my epilepsy drug needs. Dad was there when he said that I wanted to kill myself and Dad just shook his head at the flipping idiot. I diplomatically pointed out that they knew jack-shit about epilepsy and if they knew anything about it a person might say anything in the post-ictal phase (that's the post seizure phase when your mind is pretty much still scrambled).

16.   An E person needs to live in a group home or psychiatric outpatient home, all rights taken away, all financial control taken away, all anti-epilepsy-drug control taken away. One thing, I've lived independently for 19 and 1/2 years in an actual low-income senior's disabled apartment building. At age 54 I have seniority in the building meaning that I have rented there the longest. The next person down I think is around 10 years. Psychogenic (psychiatric) seizures are

tricks of the mind, sometimes attention-getting fake seizures. My seizures that have been uncontrolled for 43 years have a physical cause and not a psychiatric one. I am in control of my life, my financial, my Internet, my writing, my medical, my medication, living independently and in a future Zen Life Lesson I explain why I absolutely refuse to get a Social Worker—good intentions—in my opinion on the lower rung of the food chain ladder. I won't go on Food Stamps either as that requires you to get a Social Worker and I will not get one. I realize that a lot people get Food Stamps and more power to them, I'm not stuck up because I know that some people need that help on a monthly basis, I think that the amount is $16 each month which doesn't sound like much but it's like stocks and bonds, if you invest and let your money sit, it will grow. If you save it in five months you've got almost $100 to spend on food. I've seen at the grocery store and there are people that are using food stamps that never should have gotten them in the first place.

17. I've fired a pistol once in my life but I won't do it again as I might go into a seizure, lose consciousness and fire it at anybody from Doc P to Mom and to Dad. Talk about worst-case scenario. I also won't carry a pocket knife because in a seizure I carved up 2 very nice pillboxes and wrecked a pair of jeans. I don't handle knives if at all possible because my balance is such from being on the high powered drugs when I walk I lurch and stumble. I don't want to impale myself like a butterfly pinned to a pinning board.

18.   Epileptics—and I really do not like that word—should be run out of the country with other less than agreeable persons. I don't believe that discrimination should exist at all, no matter whom, no matter where, no matter when, and no matter why. Race and religion are irrelevant. Epilepsy doesn't care if you're male or female, gay or straight, fat or thin, exotic-dancer turquoise eyed, hazel-green eyes, have all your teeth, have no teeth, have all your hair, are bald, Islamic, Buddhist, Judeo-Christian, Scientologist, Christian realist, Native American or Mexican or Brazilian, Canadian, English, what speech you speak from English to French, to Swahili. Epilepsy is non-discriminatory and non-judgmental. And about the male / female thing, there are 2 males for every 1 female which would be great if you were online dating.

19.   A GP can treat a person's epilepsy as well as a specialist, a neurologist, may as well put an epileptologist (a neurologist specializing in epilepsy on the list.) On one of my frequent ER visits (fortunately it has been a few years since I've taken that unpleasant ambulance ride) this particular doctor accused me of wanting to commit suicide and that he or she could take over my epilepsy drug needs. This doctor is known as a pill-pusher. Dad was there when he said that I wanted to kill myself and Dad just shook his head at the flipping idiot. I diplomatically pointed out that they knew jack-shit about epilepsy and if they knew anything about it a person might say anything in the post-ictal phase (that's the

post seizure phase when your mind is pretty much still scrambled).

20.   An E person needs to live in a group home or psychiatric outpatient home, all rights taken away, all financial control taken away, all anti-epilepsy-drug control taken away. One thing, I've lived independently for 19 and 1/2 years in an actual low-income senior's disabled apartment building. At age 54 I have seniority in the building meaning that I have rented there the longest. The next person down I think is around 10 years. Psychogenic (psychiatric) seizures are tricks of the mind, sometimes attention-getting fake seizures. My seizures that have been uncontrolled for 43 years have a physical cause and not a psychiatric one. I am in control of my life, my financial, my Internet, my writing, my medical, my medication, living independently and in a future Zen Life Lesson I explain why I absolutely refuse to get a Social Worker—good intentions—in my opinion on the lower rung of the food chain ladder. I won't go on Food Stamps either as that requires you to get a Social Worker and I will not get one. I realize that a lot people get Food Stamps and more power to them, I'm not stuck up because I know that some people need that help on a monthly basis, I think that the amount is $16 each month which doesn't sound like much but it's like stocks and bonds, if you invest and let your money sit, it will grow. If you save it in five months you've got almost $100 to spend on food. I've seen at the grocery store and there are people that are using food

stamps that never should have gotten them in the first place.

21.   This one I'm repeating because it is so lame and ignorant, In Victorian days, those brilliant people who were illuminated as much as a solar eclipse thought that epilepsy was caused by excessive masturbation. I wonder what they mean by excessive. Also that statement seems to imply that all those brilliant Victorians masturbated. If excess masturbation causes epilepsy and I've nearly had epilepsy for four and a half decades I must have pretty frequent jack-attacks, that is really an ignorant statement, masturbation causes epilepsy, wisdom as wonderful as Reagan's trickle-down economics that did not work in the slightest. Do I masturbate, that isn't the kind of question you give a single male who hasn't had a girlfriend in 27 years? Again, there's that lame implication, I really have no idea where they'd get that idea, I wrote somewhere here, "In Mental Masturbation Hibernation," if it hasn't been read yet it soon will be. I was just trying to figure out a way to justify the ludicrous. I'd better lay off the topic as it is just going to piss off Don Miller and he doesn't like to be pissed off.

22.   E people don't have the best luck at picking a sexual companion and I am not talking about Cherry not having luck picking me. As I realized it Cherry and I had several bizarre conversation, there was masturbation, online dating, and the personals section of the newspaper, blind-dates set up by well-meaning relatives, rape and sexual assault, people stalking you. Mentally, Cherry was sub 7th grade with

lots of emotional insecurities that I'm going to keep to myself. I got a t-shirt that said, "Be careful what you say, I'm a writer and it might end up in my next book. I take my material from anywhere and everywhere."

23. All epileptics—again not my favorite word—are drunken reprobates. I believe that means alcoholic assholes. Really political pundits and jack-knife Jakes, Mack the masturbator, and Alf the edgy elf, persons with mental wit dulled by the high power drugs we have to take. I had a serious booze problem from light beer to Harvey Wallbangers, no whiskey, I tried it once and it burned all the way down.. I wonder what Cherry is going to do for Sheridan and her birthday and I hope she doesn't go gonzo—she didn't exactly have control over her temperament—though I haven't identified her at all, haven't gone into our private times overly much. It was an experimental time or a sex experimental time and for all the problems she had that I'm not going to mention—the girl deserves her privacy—I suppose that I still miss her, her auburn pubic hair also. Make that dark blond pubic hair that was thick and curly. Back in the 1970s that we both came from they didn't use wax at the top of the thighs or use the pubic privacy shears. She did have a great looking body and I became well acquainted with it. It looks like I'm practicing full disclosure so I'll have to be holistically adjusted and given a caffeine enema. If you like this book then send me an email giving me permission to add you to my mailing list, to thenascarepilepsyninja@gmail.com COM I'll subscribe you to the NASCAR epi-

lepsy Ninja newsletter and you'll receive word in the future about when the podcast goes live. Also, I'll send you a PDF of The Zen of Service Dogs, Buddy, the super-hero service dog, (1-1-2000 to 1-27-2014, RIP my best friend). I will also include a clickable link that will lead you to www.amazon.com/author/Millerdon I have several books published that you might be interested in. And now I have to check if a book I uploaded to KDP is actually the one I meant, November is epilepsy awareness month so a Kindle giveaway for each of my epilepsy memoir titles. I think last year the count got all the way up to 78 which are awesome. Epilepsy: The NASCAR Epilepsy Lightning Storm within the Brain: My Personal Reflections in Time's Rear-view Mirror reached #173 in the self-help category and that means it was a member of the #200 bestseller club. Detour did have a live with unpublished changes posted on it with red letters. It only took ten minutes to correct that. Now, the latest version is on there. Last year I think I put out four, make it six all total with EM40 and Detour versions of the epilepsy memoir. I wonder what Martin Colton is writing now. Maybe another cat and rat romance for all I know. It is after midnight, pills next and then bed.

24. E people are drug addicts, not in the traditional drug-abusing sense. I've called myself a legal addict and really been read the riot act. We the E have to take pills that knock us on our butts and knocks our minds out of kilter.

25. E people are not sexual beings like everyone else, Cherry sure is and maybe I flatter myself but Cherry must

have thought that Don was an okay kind of lover. I'd say that we both were sexual beings. It appears that after the split she continued being a sexual being. Only, it was a solo-sexual being. I've never been a judgmental person and I'm cool with her intimate touching herself. If she feels she needs that kind of relief it's okay with me only don't call me the next time you get loaded—I'm not sure if she's on the wagon or not—and discuss your sex life or lack of a sex life or solo sex life with me. I've heard enough from you young lady although it would be a 51-year-old lady. I don't deal well with confrontation anymore. You definitely had some confrontational days didn't you. All in all I hope she's doing well up there in Hickerson County. I'll call it lame myself if I said she still remembered who I was, she posts very little on Facebook and I can't remember the last time—if any—she personal messaged me. What she has to realize is that I'm a changed man and she isn't the reason anymore. It looks like more Cherry slams. Try—accidentally—getting punched in the balls a few times. Either it actually was an accident or I'd pissed her off. It was really easy to anger her. Just how in heck did I go off on that tangent? It is midnight so bed and now. First thing though is my pills.

26.   Just because we have epilepsy does not mean we can't think for ourselves, I suppose that's sort of like E people are stupider than other people. Sometimes the drugs we are forced to take eliminates or diminishes our intellect.

27.   Epilepsy is known as the hidden disability or hidden handicap because unless you told them or they witnessed a

seizure they'd never know that something was slightly different with their brain function. We the E are no different than other people, we live, we love, we have sex, we breathe, and we bleed just like everyone else.

28.   Epilepsy is a contagious disease. First off, epilepsy is not a disease, it is a collection of symptoms for a chronic seizural condition of the central nervous system.

29.   Epilepsy is too costly and E people should all be killed; I'm more than a little distressed at that myth. The thought that because my brain is a little different I should be removed from this world like in a Nazi death camp. Jewish and Polish, Czechs, Gypsies, blind people, persons with rheumatoid arthritis, people twisted by scoliosis, smart people and mentally diminished, I wonder how many E people were killed in the death camps, I forgot homosexuals—lesbians and male gay—no matter what color your skin was, what your theology was, what disease you had, what your politics were, what your eye-color and hair color was they killed them all. That's everyone, good, bad, or indifferent. Is that an actual myth, if it's something bad enough to give you nightmares and panic attacks I'd call that a real myth.

30.   Epilepsy is a pre-existing condition. It took a lot of campaigning and lobbying over decades to get epilepsy off the pre-existing condition list of insurance companies. It appears that it might get on it again according to the future healthcare bill.

31. Epilepsy should be removed from the ADA—Americans with Disabilities Act—list. Back in the 1990s there was that threat. The Epilepsy Foundation of America with its legal branch quashed that idea.

32. Epilepsy is not real. My reality for 54 years, 43 if we're talking E years has been that epilepsy is real because it has occupied the majority of my life—4/5—but I live, I work, I love, I breathe and I bleed just like anyone else.

33. We should be afraid of epilepsy and hide when epileptic is in sight because if we touch them we might catch their contagious epileprosy. The reason I've written different epilepsy memoirs is to educate the ignorant, you should know what something is before being frightened.

34. E people like chilling out in the nude.

35. E ladies are pretty damn sexy.

36. Make that nude and damn sexy E ladies accompanied by nude and handsome E men. And virginity is the price that we the E must pay because we shouldn't be allowed to have sex with others or ourselves.

Self and mental love requires trusting and self-trust requires honesty. I can honestly say that I hope this book helps you love yourself, the spiritual and the physical, the religious and the sexual, love your life and love yourself, and trust in the inner you, and have the courage and honesty to say that, "This is my life. I won't let a little thing like epilepsy get in the way of all my dreams and aspirations, all those goals I've kept to myself. I think all of us keep a little something to ourselves. So hop onto the excessive static-electricity roadmap, and have one hell of a ride.

Don't worry, I'm not going into my sexuality and what occurs in private or for that matter what does not occur in private, in times with me. That is no one's business but my own, just know that I'm happy with life and I guess that's the important thing to me and to others I'd think, no matter what. I've chosen celibacy and yes, virginity, there the dread confession is out, a 54 year old virgin. That reminds me of that movie back in the 1970s or possibly 1980s I think, middle-aged virgin or maybe I've got the title wrong. I'm not afraid of being a virgin and all it entails. It means that I've never had sex or protected sex with a woman or with a man.

EPILEPSY, THE OTHER E WORD

I stepped into the plastic void

No sight, no sound, no thought, no words

No memory, what does it serve

I've tried not to be annoyed, Doctors had promised that:

At the end of adolescence your seizures will stop

Like my excess brain electricity was a criminal and the doctor, a cop

I'm 53 years old now, and no longer a boy

My life has been reality; now I write and am self-employed

We take our meds day in, day out

We ask what life was all about

Some stare with pity, others shame

And think that they're somehow to blame

We pray to God, silent appeal

His is the power; physicians heal

Millions of people walk with me

The common bond: epilepsy

Don S. Miller COPYRIGHT 1975, rev. 2015

That type of complex-partial is very similar to the ones I currently have, although now I might have clusters (groupings of multiple seizures) that might last as long as an hour.

THE LIGHTNING STORM WITHIN

The lightning storm within

Oh please God not again

A loss of conscious thought

Control is lost, then sought

This is all a dream

I only want to scream

Caught in this nightmare

Do doctors even care?

The lightning storm within

Oh please god not again

I hang my head and cry

I've often wondered why

Put not your trust in God

Said the doctor who plays God

Put your trust in drugs

I only trust in love

The lightning storm within

Oh please God not again

Neither woman nor a man

Is free from seizure's chains

An electrical refrain

That plays music in my brain

Conducted by a madman

Then am I truly sane

Then I met a lady doctor

Who talked the talk and walked the walk,

We've tried for 25 years to quiet

My internal electric alarm clock

And now upon my chest it jolts

With high tech wizardry

A VNS corrects my circuits

With small bursts of electricity

My mental health suffered & my psyche broke

Schizophrenia, panic attacks, & depression so bad I rarely spoke

My harsh life's buffer chemical, daily I take

My mind, a cluttered garden, Risperdal was the rake

I've had epilepsy four decades strong

And counseled E people so they'd get along.

So Males and Females could feel they belong

I've run E Support Groups online and off

I set them straight when they tried to mouth off

Marital advice, drug recommendations

Job harassment help, private conversations

I won't have sex with a woman

And live my life in celibacy

Rather than have a defective baby

That would not make it through infancy

Don S. Miller COPYRIGHT 2012

This was written by a bitter, angry, unenlightened young man in his late 40s; it has been dedicated to my neurologist of 23 years: Patricia E. Penovich, MD, a woman who truly was compassionate about her patients, loves them, and gives a damn about what they are doing, where they are coming from in life, and fights as best she can for better seizure control for them.

GLOSSARY OF EPILEPSY TERMS

TYPES OF SEIZURES

Absence—more commonly known as 'petit mal'

Atonic—also known as a 'drop seizure' I have a partial seizure that in many ways mimics an Atonic, see Superman Seizures below

Complex-partial—also known as TLE or temporal lobe Epilepsy. My own seizures are located in the right frontal lobe, FLE: frontal lobe epilepsy, complex partials just like the temporal lobe people.

Gelastic—also known as laughing seizures (although, there is nothing funny about them)

Grand—means big, petit - means little

Mal—means sick (so grand mal means big sick, petit mal means little sick, not too helpful)

Psychomotor—another name for Complex-partial

Reflex—a seizure experienced as a reaction to some outer stimuli, possibly noise or flickering lights, television or video games

Superman Seizures—not sure of the technical name for these as Doc Penovich never said, rather than suffering ataxia—loss of control in a major muscle group—the thighs and butt just muscles just give out, in a 'Superman Seizure' my thigh muscles contract and butt muscles contract so I'm launched up and out to land with a crash. I was a runner in my youth so I have good muscles in my legs and butt and I fly a considerable distance before touching down with a thud.

Tonic-clonic—more commonly known as a 'grand mal' seizure

EPILEPSY WORDS

AED—anti-epilepsy-drug, it is also known by the term—meds, old terminology—anticonvulsant

Aura—a brief warning before a seizure occurs, this might be a sensation, a taste, a smell, a sound; I have never had the good fortune to have an aura, although for 11 years I had a seizure or sensitive detection dog that acted as a canine aura for me, letting me know ahead of time when a seizure was going to occur.

E—short for epilepsy, as a single letter is less intimidating than the whole word, we are the E people—if someone questions you, you can say the extra-special or extraordinary people

epilepsy—that's epilepsy with a small E as people diagnosed don't like putting more value on the word than there is—plain and simple—epilepsy is excess static electricity in the brain, shocking isn't it? And people can get really uptight about a little extra juice in the generator.

Epileptologist—a neurologist that specializes in Epilepsy

Marijuana—cannabis sativa (in medicinal marijuana—cannabis oil, CBD)

Neurologist—a doctor that specializes in nerves, my own specialist, Doc Penovich, is a neurologist

Neuro-surgery—surgery done on the brain

CATEGORIES

Generalized—occurring all over the brain, and thus all over the body

Partial—excess electrical activity occurring in only part of the brain

EPILEPSY-SPECIALIST ORGANIZATIONS

MEG, PA—Minnesota Epilepsy Group, Professional Associates, my current specialty group, founded by Doctor John Gates in 1990 and still going strong. My current neurologist—Patricia E. Penovich was introduced to me by Doctor Gates in 1992, when she joined the staff of the organization

MINCEP—Minnesota Comprehensive Epilepsy Program, was a patient there until 1990, still in existence, founded by Doctor Robert Gumnit and Doctor John

A Shame-free Epilepsy Memoir

Don S. Miller

Milepost 1—A Detour From the "Normal Life"

Gentlemen, Line Up Your Cars, Start Your Engines, Green Flag, Gun Your Engines, Go Go Go!

Genesis of the epilepsy, the beginning of the Electric Highway and the ups and downs of epilepsy, depression, and paranoid schizophrenia:

Noble Jameson, my first neurologist, said "I've seen this many times before. When adolescence ends, your seizures will stop." My seizures will stop when adolescence ends; that was seven or eight years; seven years seemed a lifetime, eight years seemed an eternity. So began the mounting frustration and exasperation. That statement has echoed in my mind during a 40-year prolonged adolescence. The brain is like a car's engine—it controls what we do and where we go and some of us have faulty electrical systems. In adolescence, testosterone shifted my brain into overdrive and flicked the seizure switch that controlled the firing of my spark plugs to the off position—it has remained there for over four decades. At the end of my sixth-grade-year during the hot summer of 1974 my engine overheated and I had two tonic-clonic—known at the time as grand mal—seizures. At the time I experienced ictal (seizure) amnesia. So began a 42-year-journey on Epilepsy's Electric Highway.

The fictitiously named Noble Jameson died in 2007 of liver cancer.

Memories of events prior to that time became vague and uncertain—except for certain notable exceptions. In third grade, my crush on Wendy—a redheaded, emerald-eyed girl—and in fourth, fifth, and sixth grades, Sarah—a sapphire-blue-eyed blonde, with perfect teeth who filled my thoughts and dreams.

Double Vision in the Fun House and the Wild Carnival Ride of Life

The first drug I was put on was Tegretol (carbamazepine), it had absolutely no effect in controlling my seizures—it gave me double vision (diplopia), and ringing in the ears (tinnitus). I was then put on Dilantin (sodium phenytoin), the third drug used to treat seizures—first-bromides, second-phenobarbital, third-Dilantin—the tonic-clonic seizures stopped. I was referred to Noble Jameson. They progressed to absence—then known as petit mal—and to complex-partial Epilepsy. He put me on Depakene (valproic acid), a fairly new drug at the time, it was released to the public about the time I was officially diagnosed, and Mebaral (mepho-barbital) in addition to the Dilantin. They used to use bromides for sleeping powders; it is no wonder that it turned you into a zombie.

Depakene was a terrible drug, it was in gel cap form and if the coating dissolved in your mouth there was a horrendous taste. If a pill should get stuck in your throat, it burned and you had to drink lots of water to wash it down.

I call Mebaral the zombie drug. In your liver, Mebaral is converted to phenobarbital. Everything was slowed down, thought, movement, speech. In the morning before school, my mother had to shake me awake; even then I'd fall asleep at the kitchen table. School grades suffered—going from an A in the first quarter to a D in the fourth quarter.

Dilantin was a great drug for controlling seizures, but it had an unpleasant side-effect—gingival hyperplasia—gum overgrowth. Gums would grow to the point that—in some cases—they actually covered the teeth. Then you would have to have your gums cut back by the dentist using a "La-surge" (a scalpel that cauterized the gum tissue as it sliced through).

Having had my gums cut back three times my only vivid memory of it was the smell of burned human flesh. Brush your teeth at least twice a day and floss regularly unless you want to enjoy that smell yourself.

Dilantin also decreases the free testosterone in your system, so males can have a lowered sex drive and difficulty in get-ting and keeping an erection. I haven't had that particular difficulty.

For some strange reason, women may grow mustaches and sideburns, their tender skin toughens, and their features become masculine. Being a man, I haven't inquired if this af-fects breast growth or not, though I'd guess not. But, it is a highly effective drug—I've been on it for as long as I've had Epilepsy—and I'm not knocking its ability to control Epilepsy. It wasn't until June of 2013 that I got off of Dilantin, more on that in MILEPOST 10—Stoplight at the End of the Tunnel.

I am now on a combination of Fycompa (perampanel); Briviact (brivaracetam)and generic Lamictal (lamotrigine). There is an addition, a drug called Fycompa (perampanel), it is the most expensive drug I've been on: $11 for 2 mg. I am currently taking 14 mg at bedtime, with no side effects: dizziness or funky thoughts. Quite honestly I didn't think there was such a thing as seizure free, that had occurred when on the Sabril drug study but at the cost of your eyesight, no way. I will always have abnormal brainwaves no matter what level of seizure control is achieved. I am not controlled yet I live an independent life as I hope you do, or are allowed to.

A Detour from Life, A Road Map We're Lost On

In the 1960s I was a Shelby Mustang, sleek and stylish, a racing machine; in the 1970s that Mustang transformed into a Plymouth Duster at best, a rusty, dented, surface-scratched Plymouth Duster, not too bright in his headlights. Over the years my body, mind, and brain have morphed into the poor man's muscle car—a Plymouth Duster, polished and primed for the road with a nitro supercharged engine (brain)—great speed but the gas mileage really sucks, have to use more and more of those blasted fuels—drugs—to control my seizures. I have since morphed into the Mercedes Benz F 015 driverless luxury car; still, I'm a car with an electrical system that keeps my neurologist—Patricia Penovich, very busy. As I try new fuel mixtures, I'm still liable to give a bumpy ride, and when the warning lights or indicators go on, my spark plugs fire unevenly in a staccato rhythm. Yes, life is a road map, and it takes many unforeseen twists and turns. I've been on this particular strange detour for 42 years, a road that seems to extend on, nonstop into the horizon.

Disabled people seem to run into more road signs—Stop, Slow Ahead, Rough Road, No Passing, Buckle Up and Live, Wrong Way, Drunk Drivers Will be Ticketed, Curve in Road Ahead, Yield, and hopefully not—Dead End. There is one chapter that I yanked from the book after a negative reaction from the proofreader. Its title was Slippery When Wet, something about the danger of naked showering in the night around midnight or I think it might have been stripping naked and walking the halls at night. Had that happened it would have meant eviction from Crexway but can't bloody well happen now as they have surveillance cameras in the halls now. Supposedly, it is standard practice in all HUD buildings and it is safer for insurance liability. All I know is that there are four other apartments, two of which are HUD buildings and no one else has cameras. The cameras are supposed to have cost five grand at a minimum but that is really only a guess. Maybe they think that we naked dirty dance or have group sex or masturbate until we're bruised in public. That, or will all be arrested for indecent exposure for public nudity or public masturbation. No such activity occurs in public, phrased that wrong, I don't masturbate in public or private, that's no good, worst case scenario, I think I'll just drop the subject before I put my naked foot in my mouth. That sounded a bit awkward too. My body is so beaten up and scarred up I wouldn't like to show it off... I'm off on some weird sexuality tangent. I say this later in the book, my days of being a GQ or posing nude for Playgirl are over, and that's taking another weird tangent. Virginia Cherry Stovington, as hot in temperament as hot in sexual desires taught me how to naked dirty-dance and I taught her how to French kiss, a more than equitable trade. Cherry decided that she didn't like French-kissing so we stopped. It was she that taught me the meaning of certain baseball terminology, first base was kissing, second base was breast massage, third base was mutual masturbation, home plate was intercourse, I think she thought I'd always be triple A and would never would qualify for the pros as I kept hitting pop flies and struck out a lot and seldom hit more than a double. Often, I'd get out in a squeeze play between bases. I wonder if that is too much full disclosure. That was a really weird paragraph, just how did that happen, oh, yeah, surveillance cameras, exhibitionism, masturbation. Cherry really enjoyed naked dirty-dancing or slow-dancing, she was a real music aficionado and could dance some really fancy bare footwork. She was a beautiful red-haired—maybe—girl with coarse black pubic hair that grew in 100 different directions at the same time. Occasionally we'd check just what direction it was growing. And just how did you know that information Donald Scott Miller, our kissing sessions were very visual. I definitely know that was too much full disclosure. She knew that my chest-hair at the time was red and I was a true red-haired man. She also knew that my hair was curly and it still is. Rather than claiming true memories occurred I write by the fraction principle. Part fact (maybe) and part fiction (maybe) = FRACTION, FRACTION = REALISTIC EPILEPSY FICTION. Possibly I mention this in the book, on one of my frequent ER visits in 2013 I was given a naked MRI and got a letter from Doctor Reginald Smyth your brain shows signs of atrophy, possible chronic anticonvulsant use, really, yeah, I guess that 39 years of anti-epilepsy-drug use would be chronic. Then, the kicker, skull malformations show symptoms of Pie's disease or osteoblastic metastatic syndrome. That, by the way is bone cancer. I don't remember as well as I used to and sometimes forget entirely. Doc Penovich consulted a radiologist familiar with my case, it's nothing to worry about, and the so called skull malformations are merely from prolonged Dilantin use.

My ramblings continued...

And, by disabled, I mean persons having Epilepsy. We, the E people, 1% to 3% of the World population, taking the 2% median, in the USA—approximately—6 million people, 4 million males, 2 million females; or, in the total World population, approximately—139 million people, 92.5 million males, 46.5 million females. That is a substantial number of people, many of whom are driving the road alone, tired, and afraid.

I have fictionalized names of classmates, support group members, some doctors—namely, my first neurologist and some other notables, but have used the real names of Patricia Penovich, MD, John Gates, MD, and Robert Gumnit, MD, Robert Meisterling, MD, and Nicholas Weiss, MD. Mr. John Stohr is the name of an actual person.

Got No Dents On Me

Saint Croix Central Junior High and High School, Wisconsin, USA

Foggy Road Ahead and Potential Car Wreck

No Room In The Parking Lot For The New City Kid

In 1975, we moved from Stillwater, Minnesota to Hammond, Wisconsin. I was a city kid confronted not only with dealing with my seizure condition but also with classmates who for the most part were farm-kids. I hadn't been born there, so I was always considered an outsider.

In 1975—I attended one quarter of 7th grade at Stillwater Junior High, I remember Herr Spreeman was the German language teacher. We moved to a small town in Wisconsin, and I had small town culture shock. You could easily have fit five of the small public library building into the Stillwater Public Library building.

The first day I attended Junior High School there I did not make a good impression. I walked with the bouncing city strut I'd grown up with. Being the new kid that knew all the answers did not make me 'Mister Popularity.'

In Mister Larsson's Human Events class, someone passed a note to me, it was from a girl—Cindy Landon. She wanted to know if I wanted to be 'boyfriend/girlfriend?' I had this cockiness, city-kid superiority thing going on and without even asking who she was, I said 'No.' Little did I know that Cindy was the prettiest girl in the 7th, 8th, 9th, the whole high school for that matter. All through high school I kicked myself. I had a crush on her from the moment I saw who she was back in 7th grade through my one year at UW-RF (University of Wisconsin - River Falls). I still find her the most beautiful woman I've ever met and called friend.

Soon, I did have a girlfriend, Desiree, mostly because at that point we were the two most intelligent people in 7th grade. Considering the amount of meds I was on this doesn't say much for the scholastic level of the small town educational system. Desiree was my girlfriend in 7th and 8th, and then we hit the big time, we were in high school. In my freshman and sophomore years of high school, I had no girlfriend.

Bumper to Bumper Touch, Almost

Both Desiree and I had noses that were larger in size than other people. One Friday night, behind an old school bus, I tried to kiss her, actually we tried kissing but as my Grandpa Fred might have put it, 'we bumped beaks,' and I ended up kissing the corner of her mouth. That was pleasurable, but not what I'd intended, or what she'd expected, and it wasn't much longer and we broke up, for good. If I'd had a second chance, well, that was a long time ago and the calendar pages don't flip backwards. I was a shy boy and it took a year and a half to get the courage to give Desiree a little smooch. Is youth the time of greatest happiness, or greatest vulnerability? That's a Hercule Poirot quote (Agatha Christie).

Small-town Girl Games, the Tilt-a-Whirl, and Spin until You Drop

In my junior and my senior year, I had a girlfriend—Roberta Beltier who had flawless skin, except when she had a bad case of poison ivy from the class one year below me, or was it two, sorry, it's been over three decades. During my senior year I tutored a well-developed freshman girl named Samantha Sykes-Fairbairn in mathematics and she taught me how to French Kiss, more than an equitable trade. One guy plus one girl divided by hundreds of kisses equal two happy people with smiles on their faces. Our separate lanes didn't merge in a head-on collision, thankfully, or if you prefer, we never locked front bumpers and revved our engines to the tango beat, I was 17 and 18 and she was let's see—15, I had no intention of getting a count of statutory rape against me.

Samantha's algebra grades didn't make a drastic improvement, and why had they picked me, my math grades really stunk? Call it conceit, but I think I was a direct request from a freshman girl who wanted to prove to her friends she could take a senior boy away from a junior or sophomore girl. Roberta was a pig farm-girl that lived miles away, in the country. Samantha Sykes-Fairbairn was a townie like me and her house was just a five-minute walk across town; Samantha had a distinct advantage. I think there was more than a little friction between town and country factions.

Roberta and I had a roller-coaster relationship with more lows than highs, that lasted through my one checkered year of college, and then she discovered another way to get high, someone had introduced her to Mary Jane, weed, grass, pot, roach, reefer or any of the other nicknames for marijuana. I tried it once, way back when, but it didn't do anything. It was just as well as I had enough neurological problems—I didn't need a brain made of tapioca pudding.

The Wonders Of The Wicked Weed, Medicinal Marijuana, Cannaboid Oil In The Wildly Racing Engine

As long as we're talking about marijuana, they have something called 'medicinal marijuana' to treat seizures now—cannaboid oil—cannabadiol. Call me square or uptight, maybe time has made my attitudes as intractable as my seizures. If the seizures are that bad and you are drug-resistant, then I can see it. I am not inflexible in the way I view things, I saw too many people whose brains rotted away from using Mary Jane, perhaps time has made my atti-tudes as intractable as my seizures are. Doc Penovich, my neurologist of 23 years gave her candid opinion. She said in some cases, emphasis on some it worked in children—about a 10% efficacy rate, or it worked for one in 10 people. She shared a little tidbit—smoking it won't do it—so don't start, if it did she'd have several patients seizure free. She didn't breach confidentiality because she didn't name names. Before the appointment you are given two sheets—one is for psychiatric stuff, the other, list your medical rec-ord since the last appointment; in the space—Do you use recreational drugs? They'd checked the yes box and listed Mary Jane after Names?

You Are Not Alone

I promised honesty in the introduction and I'm giving it to you. In the fall of 1978—my sophomore year something happened I have to mention so you'll know—no matter what your age or sex that you aren't the only one. Mister Pe-terson, a really cool guy, English teacher, and I were talking in the front of his classroom, as it had filled up with fresh-man students. I had a seizure and was incontinent (pissed my pants). I got exceptionally embarrassed, as in humiliat-ed, and ended up walking across town to home, to change. I remember being so embarrassed, that I stayed home for the rest of the day. I don't believe my parents were even aware of it at the time.

This happened three times that quarter (same scenario, same classroom). Walking the halls, I could hear the snickers behind me, the whispering and talking behind hands. Had it been my class, things might have been cool, but these were younger boys and girls and harassment was a break from the daily monotony of education. Sorry about using the word—cool, but I am a child of the 1970s.

After having a seizure in public, during gym class, things changed—when playing softball, I wasn't allowed to play in the field, and for some reason, not bat. I could only play catcher for both teams—a position no one else wanted. Not only did I have to play catcher, I also had to play ref or umpire, calling balls and strikes, and no one likes a zebra—a referee and those black bars on the zebra's hide became like prison bars to me. I remember there being both boys and girls, then again, it was a long time ago. Wrestling was just boys as it would have been a little awkward if certain body parts had begun to develop and judging by girlfriends I had the hormone estrogen was in full swing.

In 1973, pre-the E thing, I did wrestle with a male, sixth grade classmate named Chris something, just like I was a word I hate—normal. From 1974 on, things changed fast; wrestling was a physical contact sport. Don might strike his head and you know what might happen then, plus the district might be liable for damages. So, it was write a paper—1000 word minimum—on wrestling in the library. That took all of a half hour, so I spent my time checking out the bookshelves and found the females in the library far more interesting than the males in the gym class.

A King Day-mare and Nightmare

Fright on the Dark Side

Study hall was interesting because rather than study we had marathon card games of UNO. A senior girl named Opal Juarez loaned me a book that would change my life. It was the second of Stephen King's—Salem's Lot. It was like Dracula, set in small town America—Jerusalem's Lot, Maine. I have to tell you that every time I read it, I get out a cross or crucifix, it scares me that much. Now I have the Salem's Lot audiobook on my MP3 player—I downloaded it off of Youtube and converted the video to an MP3 using Any Video Converter—freeware edition.

In 1979, "Salem's Lot," the movie, starring David Soul and Bonnie Bedelia, aired on TV. That movie really freaked me out; scared the Be-jeezus out of me and Mister King has managed to do that all my life. In 2004, an updated Salem's Lot, with Rob Lowe in David Soul's role—the writer, Ben Mears, aired on TNT. Rutger Hauer played the head vampire—Mister Kurt Barlow. The time-line was shifted from the 1970s to after one of the Gulf Wars. I know because I was at the CCC—Continuing Care Center, a nursing home recovering from a seizure-related fracture of my right ankle—August 1, 2004, to Halloween, October 31, 2004, and caught only part of it.

I got hooked on King's work and have followed the man's career for 34 years now. Long ago I decided to become a writer of dark fiction—and with Stephen King as mentor, that dream is becoming reality. Oh, by the way, Opal, after 30 years, that copy of Salem's Lot fell to pieces and I had to replace it. That was a long book loan. Opal, should I ever attend a class reunion; that is something extremely doubtful; this year, 2014 is number 33, I will have a brand new copy for you. Her name wasn't Opal, but another gemstone of a similar coloration. Her name wasn't Juarez either, but something similar in nature.

Not a Member of the Athletic Pit Crew

I joined the basketball team and that lasted one practice. We were doing lay-ups (dribble the ball, when close to the basket, jump in the air off one foot, ball bounces off the backboard, through the net, and score). The dribbling part was going pretty good, then I froze in place and the ball continued bouncing into the wall. I don't know whether that was a seizure or not; what I do know is that after that, there weren't enough uniforms, but we're glad you're in the Pep Band and we're glad you can support the team that way. You can try again next year; I never did, the way the situation had been handled left a sour taste in my mental mouth, and I'd no desire for a repeat performance of the previous year.

The golf team was made up of six Varsity and six Junior Varsity members, just mattered how low you scored during the qualifying round during the week. You could be a Junior or Senior and score 45, but if you scored higher than six other men on the team, you were on the JV team, at least for that round. There were thirteen men on the team; for four straight years I was thirteenth man. This had nothing to do with Epilepsy, just that I was a poor athlete and had what I call a buttonhook slice. Relatively speaking, I'm tall—five-foot, eleven and three-quarters inches, never got that extra quarter inch to call it six foot and have long gorilla arms. At the time I had horrendous coordination. The small town in which we lived had a golf course and starting in seventh grade, with a set of mismatched clubs, graduating eventually to a matched set of Delta clubs, I played golf as best I could.

However, my drive would leave the T-box straight and it would begin curving so far to the right that distance-wise, the ball actually appeared to be heading back toward me. I could go to the golf course before they opened, at 7:00 am on a Saturday morning, by me—hit drives perfectly straight and one or two putt. Put me with two or more people and my game fell apart. It's a sad state of affairs when your divot—clump of grass travels farther than your ball. Either that or you strike only air and look down the fairway for your ball that had to have gone a mile, you hit it so perfect, you didn't even hear it hit the club-head face. Then, reality strikes, as you look down and the ball is still sitting on the tee, waiting for you. Oh, that still counts as one stroke.

I finally straightened that slice out by combining my swing with a power-draw, and became an awesome chipper negating some of the bad strokes I still hit, and then I had ACL-Reconstruction surgery, no rotational movement in that knee anymore, so my golfing days and hopes of going professional ended.

I Don't Drive, Honey

I've never had a driver's license and have no desire to get one. In my senior year, the spring of 1981, I learned the hard way about the opposite sex's opinion of that was. The Prom was coming up and like anyone else I wanted to attend with someone in my own class. I approached three of the girls in my class about going, who we'll call Lacey, Tracey, and Stacey, and this is a direct quote, "Uh, uh, no way. I 'd have both hands on the wheel and you'd have two hands free," repeated three times, each about an hour apart, I don't think there was a conspiracy but it was a curious mindset for these three women to have back in the not-so-innocent—1970s and early 1980s. Lacey was striking and had long straight black hair, brown eyes, and perfect teeth, a product of an orthodontist's braces. The other two definitely weren't beauty contest contestants.

That was hard to take when at the beginning of my adolescence, according to Noble Jameson. Just what kind of sexual stories about me were going around? When did Don—the divot-digger—become Lester—the molester, or Gary—the groper? I could have taken Samantha to the dance, we both lived in town and could have walked there together, as Roberta was battling through a bout with 'poison-ivy face,' but I wanted to take out someone the same age as I was, and would have really been razzed by fellow classmates, female and male, for taking a freshman girl to Prom. As far as taking a girl out to eat, I had this 'not being able to drive' thing that hung around me like a foul smell, and we've already heard the opinions of three female classmates—Lacey, Tracey, and Stacey, "Uh, uh, no way..."

I went stag—alone and walked across town to the gym, stayed for one dance, then walked home, my disco pumps clocking on the road surface. This is going to really age me, but I was wearing a light-blue leisure suit. I think leisure suits were revenge for some less than reputable fashion designers. I honestly don't know what became of Samantha and Roberta, just that there was exceptional dislike between the two of them, thanks to me no doubt.

Teacher: John Stohr's Tragic Death

This was 1979, my junior year in high school, before the ADA—the American's With Disabilities Act that protects the rights of disabled persons. A wonderful teacher named John Stohr, left his position and met a tragic end.

After having had two grand mal seizures in a classroom in late 1979, he received an official call telling him he'd have to vacate his teaching position—School Board members never realized the finality of that statement or pretended not to. I'm not naming names, but John was fired because he had E and had the misfortune to have a couple seizures in public where students could see. Early in 1980, he began working for a major newspaper in the Twin Cities of Minnesota—Saint Paul and Minneapolis—as regional delivery manager. He died tragically in a fiery, seizure-related auto accident. John Stohr, a man I called both teacher and friend (1948 – 1980). That is only 32-years-old, now, at age 52, I realize just how young that is. His being fired and his death are a matter of public record, I'm not making anything up, it actually happened.

Ethanol in the Fuel Tank

Alcohol Abuse and Addiction

Introduction to Fuel Additives

First, I want to say that I'm not proud of what happened, but it is reality, it all occurred. And I promised you honesty so here it is, bared to the bones. Life can lead you onto some really strange roads. I want to emphasize that I do not want to preach to you—Thou Shall Not; I just want you to know if you're on the same road there are people more than willing to help you. Contact your school counselor or check out the ads in the newspapers or Yellow Pages.

The first time I got drunk was the fall of 1978, my sophomore year of high school. At the time I was an alcohol virgin, I had little drinking experience to draw back on. In the fall of this year, that is 36 years ago. I was a member of the High School Pep Band—attending a football game—and had returned my tuba to the band room. I noticed that some of the cheerleaders had red noses, rosy cheeks, and you could tell by the fumes they were breathing out that something wasn't kosher. They were also sipping from their lip-gloss bottles; somehow, they had managed to fill them with whiskey.

At half time, the cheerleaders all disappeared, and my friend Stanley S. said, "C'mon, Don, it's party time!"

We drove over to Twin Lakes, really not much more than two puddles in a farmer's field outside a nearby town. Big Mike, a large-sized man who had graduated two years previously came over not long after we'd arrived. Big Mike had a police scanner walkie-talkie hung on his belt and was nephew of one of the town cops so we knew we were safe as kittens to get hammered.

He was drinking a can of Mountain Dew. He poured half of its contents onto the ground, pulled a pint of blackberry brandy out of his pocket, and poured it into the Mountain Dew can, filling it three-quarters full. Shaking it a little to mix the two elements, he handed it to me. It was one noxious cocktail, but after I started drinking it, in a little while I didn't notice the taste anymore. Everything became extremely funny and people and the surroundings began to move in slow motion, then spin—this was my first experience with chemical-induced escapism and it was not all pleasant—in time I grew to like the feeling of not being in control. Both Stanley and Big Mike are now deceased—Big Mike from excess weight, Stanley S., from unknown causes. In respect, both will remain nameless as far as their actual names; people who went to Saint Croix Central know full well the identities of Stan and Mike, how the former had been labeled an agitator and troublemaker, then made good, serving Uncle Sam overseas.

Highway to Hell

The next morning I discovered that there was a price to be paid. I never had a hangover in my life, but it felt as if a giant hand had taken hold of my legs and another my chest and proceeded to wring me out like a washrag. After the initial vomiting, the dry heaves commenced. My abdominal muscles were sore to the touch. This was the first time I prayed to the porcelain goddess, head hung over the toilet bowl, puking, or at least attempting to. Needless to say my parents were not pleased. I thought to myself, only an idiot would make a repeat of last night and this morning.

The next football game was in a town far to the south of us, it was a repeat performance—this continued during the football season, town after town, game after game. This was over 30 years ago and laws pertaining to liquor were loosely enforced—sorry to tell law enforcement that, but it was all too true, I'd say one third of my high school class, maybe as high as 80%, had a serious problem with alcohol.

Wisconsin's baseball team is the Milwaukee Brewers—need I say more. If I had a beer, the old inhibition switch was turned to the off position. So yes, I had a serious problem with alcohol—time has magnified, rather than diminished that in my memory.

In the Good Old Summertime

I'd graduated high school at this point in time, and I was lying back in my room cutting some Zs. A man named Pete—from my class drove his Dad's convertible, and pulled up in front of our house on the eastern edge of town. He knocked on the front door, it was a weekend, Good Neighbor Days in the nearby town and the result is that we got hammered, plastered, legally stoned, green to the gills, stewed, or any of the many other idioms for intoxicated. As usual, I paid the price on Sunday morning, Church for me that day was praying to the porcelain goddess—the toilet.

A Party Town

I went to college—the University of Wisconsin, River Falls—for one year. River fall was known as a party town with eight bars—I knew the inside of several of them. When you have classes at 8:00 a.m. and 9:30 a.m. and you sleep in until 1:00 p.m. it does not do wonders for the grade-point-average. That year I blacked out two times, with the amount of prescription medication I was taking in combination with the amount of alcohol, it is a wonder I didn't end up on a slab in the morgue. My church's former Pastor, Carol Ann, said she was sure God had another purpose for me.

Country Detox

We moved to just outside of Hudson, Wisconsin, way out in the middle of nowhere, on Highway 35, 6 miles from Hudson, 8 miles from River Falls—I basically dried out. After three years of sobriety, in 1986, I began attending classes at

WITI "witty" (Wisconsin Indianhead Technical Institute)—now known as WITC (Wisconsin Indianhead Technical College) for a course called—Microcomputer Accounting Assistant. It promised to be a bad year, one in which I staggered down a twisting turning road that had a faded sign that read—Alcoholic Stupor at the roadside

A group of us went to a dinner/play at the Old Log Theater. I believe the play was called "Lights Out." At intermission, I wandered out to the bar, some instinct told me no, damned if I was going to lose control again, damned if I was going home unable to remember what I'd seen. Out of instinct I'd ordered a Light Miller Beer, I took one swallow and the taste sickened me and I knew that God had given me another purpose to live for. So, I won't preach to you.

That was in 1986, it will be 2 years since I drank any alcohol in the fall of this year, 2015. Oh, there has been the odd shot glass of communion wine, but now at Zion Lutheran—the church I belong to they have grape juice as well as the wine. My mother's side gets together on Christmas Eve and one Christmas Eve Mom thought I might like to join in and have a glass of wine with everyone else, it tasted like vinegar and I wanted to puke. My body rejected it like I was allergic to it, and I was glad. Christmas Eve, a couple years ago, we had a bottle of sparkling alcohol-free grape juice, and that's as close as I'll ever come to wine again. I have had Sharps and O'Douls non-alcohol beer that is not exactly my idea of good tasting; still, it's better than the alternative.

Milepost 2— Computerized Diagnostic Testing Of the Electrical System

Depth Electrodes Implantation

As part of a standard neurological checkup, they gave me an EEG (electro-encephalogram)—with unclear results. A seizure is abnormal spiking discharge—excess static electricity within the brain. In a generalized seizure—spiking discharge is all over the brain; the discharge from a complex partial seizure is confined to one part. The spiking discharge recorded came from all over the brain—this would normally occur during a tonic-clonic (grand mal) generalized seizure. As Doc Penovich has only recently reminded me—Donald Scott Miller—named for his dead Uncle Donald Willis Miller—does not have generalized seizures, he has partial seizures and one kind mimics an Atonic seizure. The most dramatic of those are what I call—Superman Seizures, I fly through the air, then crash land.

Looking at a past CAT scan or skull X-ray—they decided that my skull was thicker than the average person's. The skull dissipated the electrical discharge or spiking activity giving a false generalized reading. Officially and medically, they told me that I had a thick skull; that's something that I've been accused of more than once during my 40-year journey.

My neurologist at the time was Doctor Ramon Sanchez—member of the staff of—Minnesota Comprehensive Epilepsy Program—MINCEP.

Doctor Robert Boswell was to be the neurosurgeon. I was given a CAT scan of the skull; different measurements were taken in regard to skull size—top to bottom, fore to aft, and side-to-side—and entered into a "brilliant" computer program he'd designed decided placement of the depth electrodes. This was sometime in the 1980s when Apple was still growing and Big Blue was in the driver's seat. In the end, placement of the electrodes had been a bit more barbaric than I'd been led to believe.

I was shaved cue-ball-bald before surgery and fitted with a HALO—a circular piece of metal with a threaded fitting in the back. They tightened four fiberglass/plastic screws in the four "corners" of the HALO—the pressure became so intense I passed out and fell to the floor. Fortunately I didn't bust out my front teeth like I did some time in the future. HALO is also an aviation term for parachuting—high altitude low opening, you jump from such a height you need an oxygen tank, and drop like a rock, then open the chute really low down. It is supposed to be exhilarating and produce an adrenalin rush, my own personal falling HALO made one nurse realize they'd tried fitting a super-sized family of 10 into a Volkswagen Beetle. Now, that might work if you're circus performer of shorter stature, but not on a head that had a 7 5/8 Stetson hat-size A larger HALO was brought and comfortably screwed in place. They wheeled me into the operating room on a gurney and lifted my body onto the operating table.

They raised my upper body and the HALO was brought back so that it fit thread to threaded fitting. A hand screw with large knob had been turned clockwise; they tightened the joint, and locked me into place.

For proper placement of the electrodes Doctor Boswell and his surgical assistant were busy writing on my scalp. This was essential for proper placement according to the great computer diagrams I assumed they'd made. In the end, they were a bit more barbaric than high-tech in electrode final placement.

I received four injections of a substance considerably stronger than Novocain. Two—directly above my eyes, three quarters of the way up on the forehead, and two—about an inch and a half directly above and just behind the ears.

The electrodes they were going to implant were the diameter of the ball on a ballpoint pen. They were several inches in length.

I heard a roaring noise coming from within my skull as they drilled the hole. "What are you using Doctor, a Black and Decker?" I swear, absolute truth, I did ask that.

"It's called a Yankee drill, Mister Miller." The Yankee drill—hand operated, had a special bit so that it wouldn't create bone chips. Before, they sewed a black (carbon) disc in place directly over the hole they drilled as a guide.

As the first electrode slid in I endured the worst agony I had in my life up to that point. Pain radiated outward through my head. Then, finally—two times, each side of my head—the electrodes were fixed into place. Then it was time for the forehead. The pain—not as intense initially drove all thoughts from my mind. The endorphins or natural pain-killers were working overtime. As they slid the electrode home my eye shut and I saw a white light as a branding iron touched my brain.

They watched my reactions and I heard, and this is an actual quote, "Okay, we hit the optical nerve. Pull it back a centimeter." That was what they meant by computer-aided placement. Again, I swear that is what they said.

They wired me to the wall in the Intensive Monitoring Suite—IMS and two pretty, soft, and curvaceous women nurses accompanied me—one on my left, one on my right if I needed to use the bathroom. I didn't really mind. Attending to your bodily functions with an audience in attendance really sucked.

Doctor Sanchez had an irritating nickname for a seizure—pop. In the morning, he'd be making his rounds and his head would pop around the doorframe and say, "Have you popped yet?" If I hadn't he lowered my medication in the hopes of inducing a seizure. After two weeks, I felt like popping Doctor Sanchez's "Schnoz."

For three weeks after they implanted the electrodes—I didn't have a seizure. This irritated Doc Sanchez and me—as it was a diagnostic procedure to record my seizures on audio and video. About three weeks down the line I went seizure-crazy. I had one hundred forty-two complex-partial seizures one after the other—in twenty minutes. That is a new seizure every eight seconds, I was completely exhausted. According to Jenny, Doc Penovich's nurse, there is such a thing as CP status epilepticus, and that is what I was in. Then, to stop them—I was given a shot, a bolus of an AED—Depakene up the rectum. Depakene, that wonderful drug I was put on in 1974 or 1975, but it did work, the seizures stopped.

Doctor Sanchez then removed the electrodes, and here I will pause.

Time for an educational lesson—picture the brain as a lump of modeling clay the size of your two fists put together; your forearms form the spinal cord. Jam four knitting needles into it, one on each side, and two in front. When you remove the needles there are pockets of air that escape.

When Doctor Sanchez removed the electrodes, the air went around to the front of my skull and I had the worst headache I've had in my life—I assume that is what a migraine headache feels like. If I leaned forward, the pain doubled; they shot me full of painkillers. Eventually, the air escaped, possibly out of those wonderful holes they'd drilled.

My parents—Neil and Grace—and I were then part of a medical meeting with Doctor Sanchez, and Doctor Boswell. The end result of this—they told me I had dual foci, a double area where seizures started, right and left—no surgery would be possible. Another drug—Peganone (ethotoin)—a relative of Dilantin would be tried. I assumed that they'd named it after the winged horse Pegasus from Greek mythology—another dream that fell flat, or maybe I should say, splat!

At a much later time, I was told by my current neurologist—Doctor Patricia E. Penovich that the electrical disturbance originates in the right frontal lobe, and that surgery may be possible—a frontal lobectomy—however, that is not an option I'd even consider, at least at this point in my life.

Milepost 3— Canine Seizure Control (Service Dog in the Front Seat)

A Little History

The majority of this was written before 1-27-2014. Buddy's a beautiful, yellow Labrador retriever and is probably the gentlest creature on the face of the earth. He was bred and trained at Sunshine Service Dogs, Inc., in Luck, Wisconsin. Director Lori Peper-Rucks trains dogs for hearing, mobility, sensitive-detection, law enforcement, and search and rescue.

Buddy was born in January of 2000. In the first year of his life, he lived with a foster family who took the responsibility of feeding and caring for him. Beginning in his second year, he lived at Sunshine and began the intensive training needed to become a service dog.

Buddy is sponsored by the Grantsburg Animal Hospital. This means that he receives basic care free of charge, and food and medications at a special discounted rate. His vet is Doctor Pete Magnuson. Cost for dog food made me go with Purina Dog Chow, Buddy didn't seem to mind.

Those Damned Wood-ticks

In the late spring of 2003 Buddy had a bout with Lyme disease. Doctor Pete prescribed the antibiotic, doxycycline. I was supposed to give him two pills every four hours, eight pills a day. I had to give him one pill at a time, prying his jaws open, and shoving the pill as far back in his mouth as I could. Before he could work the pill forward with his tongue, I clamped my hands around his muzzle until he swallowed. He got the second pill down with no problem...I thought. Then he reared back and threw up all over the shag carpeting. He threw up six times that morning. His stomach could not handle that dose of the antibiotic at all. After talking it over with Doctor Pete, I ended up giving him one pill early in the morning and another in mid-afternoon until the pill bottle was empty. After animals have been treated for and cured of Lyme's, they will still test positive for it, for a number of years. Buddy now tests negative for it.

Early Warning System

While at a grocery store, we were headed down the aisle. Buddy was leading the way on the left side of the shopping cart. He stopped and looked over his shoulder at me. I ignored him. We went a bit further and he stopped and looked over his shoulder. I ignored him again. We went a bit further yet and he stopped, turned his body around completely, sat in front of me, and glared. If Buddy could talk, "Listen up Buster, you ignored the first two, you aren't going to miss this one." Thirty minutes later, while we were in a restaurant, I had two seizures. The first involved slipping in and out of consciousness for about ten minutes. The second lasted about fifteen minutes. I needed to learn to trust Buddy's instincts.

We spent a good deal of our initial time together learning how to read each other. Not only must he be able to sense a seizure coming, I must be able to read what he is trying to tell me.

Sensitive-Detection Dog

Buddy is a sensitive-detection dog, sometimes referred to as a "seizure dog." He is able to detect a change in smell due to an altered chemical balance that occurs in me about ten minutes before a seizure. Buddy knows what I smell like normally and is able to pick up on that change. When this happens, he attempts to let me know. This is called detection. Since Buddy was placed with me in March of 2003 he has had over three hundred detections. The Superman Seizures occur so quickly; Buddy really has no time to react to them. There's no detection, ten minutes, seizure. It's standing and fly through the air, crash land on the floor in the matter of a second or two.

Once, as we were headed across the room he stopped and began backing up into me. He forced me backward into a chair and planted himself on top of my feet. There was absolutely no chance that I could have been able to get up and move with him positioned as he was. Ten minutes later, I had a seizure.

Another time, I started to get up from the chair by the computer. Buddy stood in front of me blocking the way. First he stood on all four legs, and then he'd drop down to his forelegs, and back up again. He whined, talked, and bounced up and down. I took the hint and sat down. Shortly after I had a ten-minute seizure. There are hundreds more detections but I'm sorry to say I didn't keep a journal of them; those were a good assortment of them though.

About Service Dogs

When a Service Dog is placed with a person, it is for a probationary period of six months. At the end of that time they check to see that you've kept up with his health care, eating regimen, and exercise. The animal/handler team is then tested in various ways and if they pass, the dog becomes fully certified. Buddy was placed with me March 21st, 2003 and was fully certified September 22nd, 2003.

Placement

"I always tell our volunteers that I wish everyone could be there when I place a service dog with its new owner, they are so excited about their new partner and for the help these dogs give them. The dogs change their lives dramatically," said Peper-Rucks.

Service Dogs are People Too

One of the first things I was told before he was placed with me was not to treat him like a person. If I did so, it would really screw him up psychologically. Sometimes he acts more like a person than a dog, though.

Buddy can be a real ham. When he rolls on his back and gets his belly scratched, his lips peel back revealing all his teeth. He'll lie there with a slaphappy grin on his face that disappears only after I've finished. He also break-dances. While lying on his back, he'll curl his body into C's, wriggling left then right, dancing to a beat that only he hears.

Occasionally, Buddy will get a sheepish grin with a bit of a wolfish smirk to it. This is when he gets a case of room clearing gas. It's like a combination of sulfur and rotten cantaloupes.

One night, I was watching a DVD and enjoying a bag of microwave popcorn. Before leaving for the next room, I set the bag on the floor. Next thing, I heard "THUMP! THUMP! THUMP! THUMP!" I returned and saw that Buddy had his head stuck in the bag and it was covering his eyes. He was banging his head into the wall. When I finally pulled the bag off, I got a big thank-you slurp to the side of my face.

Buddy has a collection of stuffed animals. They all look like they've had some pretty rough treatment. His rabbit has one ear, teddy bear is minus a head, and he has a three-legged teddy dog. He likes picking them up between his teeth, throwing his head back, and letting go. Some afternoons are filled with flying rabbits, teddy bears, and teddy dogs. He loves animals that have squeakers in them. It's as though the squeaker is the prize in a Cracker Jack box. He'll chew off arms, legs, ears, or tails and pull out the stuffing to get at this "treasure."

Canine Cologne

They were also stinking up the apartment, dog breath can be bad enough to set you running to the other end of the room; for some reason, that is at the hottest time of the year and Buddy insists on hanging on me and dog slobber can really reek. Anyway, in clearing the dog stink out of my apartment, all his stuffed animals went, from his first teddy-dog, to his new pink piggy, my shag carpeting went, a lefto-ver shag remnant I'd put under my bed went, a remnant of my new carpet that was in front of the sink went. And not surprisingly, most of the dog smell went. I now have a su-per-duper Dyson vacuum that sucks up all his dog hair, and the cylinder or canister of it is always full of dog hair every time I vacuum. He's an indoor dog, almost 24/7, so, it is like the tropics and he sheds hair continually.

Buddy to the Rescue

In mid-summer of 2003 we were out walking, about two or three blocks from our apartment building and were halfway across a street. I went into a seizure that involved severe disorientation. Buddy took charge. He pulled me across that street, and another, and up a slight incline until we were in the parking lot in front of our apartment building. At that point I regained enough consciousness to realize what he'd done.

During this type of seizure I'm completely unaware of my surroundings. When Buddy led me across those two streets, it must have been like pulling a two hundred pound weight behind him. A car could easily have struck me; he really did save my life.

Afterward, Buddy got a prolonged bear hug from me. I'm not ashamed to admit it, but the fur on the back of his neck was wet with tears of gratitude.

One more time

In 2010, Buddy couldn't keep any food I fed him down, yet again. After trying repeatedly, I called the emergency weekend phone number for the Veterinarian, who at this time was Greg Palmquist. He set an early morning—about 10:00 am—appointment on Monday. They drew blood, but were shooting blanks, until Greg said, "I know he's negative now, but let's give him a Lyme disease test." He was positive. And so, he began a regimen of huge Amoxicillin tablets. He's much better now.

Buddy Miller, Hero

The WVMA (Wisconsin Veterinary Medical Association) selected Buddy to be the Wisconsin Pet Hall of Fame's 2011 Hero Inductee. So now, Buddy is officially a hero with a gold medal/blue ribbon to prove it. That summer, just after being placed with me, he truly did save my life, so it is an honor he deserved.

Buddy and the Falling Toilet Seat Lid

Buddy had been getting on some in years; it had been September 11, 2012. It was a hot day; I'd been busy writing all day and man was my eyes getting bloodshot. Stephen King says he writes every day of the year save one: Christmas. Mister King said in On Writing that he wrote every day of the year. So I guess I've been taking lessons from the master of his craft.

The day had been hot and for some reason my AC either wasn't working or it had been turned off. Buddy had drained his water-bowl three times but was still was thirsty. So he'd padded into the bathroom, stuck his nose under the seat and flipped it up in the air. He managed to get a few slurps of water before the toilet-seat lid came crashing down on his head. I heard a 'Yike' of fright then he came padding back, shamefacedly, and lay down behind me; he detected three seizures that afternoon.

Puppy Love

I'd be lost without him and I think he'd be lost without me. It's amazing how Buddy took over part of my life so completely, that love, even in its most primitive state can pass between man and beast. The Budster-doggy saved my life that time; and thanks to the miracle of antibiotics, Grantsburg Animal Hospital and I have saved his life twice.

Is There a "Dog-tor" In the House?

Some people don't believe that Buddy knows when my pill times are. At 8:00 am, 5:00 pm, and 10:00 pm Buddy will come over, sit by me, and won't leave until after I've taken my meds. That's something they couldn't have trained him for.

Buddy also knows when I'm feeling ill or depressed. At those times he'll come over and snuggle up close to me. Hugging a warm, living, breathing dog—a dog with nothing but love to give in return—can do wonders to raise your spirits.

On the Job

A Service Dog is a highly trained canine, which assists disabled people in need. As the owner of a service dog I can tell you firsthand about the changes the addition of Buddy to my life brought, he has lifted my self-esteem, boosted my ego, and broadened my horizons. Buddy enables me to overcome the obstacles life has laid in front of me. With his help I was able to locate what turned out to be only short-term work in a computer-related job and have been pursuing a personal goal of mine, creative writing. End of the Leash

Buddy Miller 01-01-2000 to 01-27-2014 was put to sleep today (01-27-2014), his kidneys had shut down, white count was high, wasn't producing red blood cells, and the Vet said everything was backing up inside. He was 14 years—98 dog years young and ready to go.

Buddy also had an occasional "grand mal" seizure and had his own prescription for phenobarbital, but I hated to use it on him. His body would experience a minor shudder. I don't know if it was a sympathetic seizure but he was awful protective of me.

There is a photo of me with my two guitars and one of Buddy in one of his break-dancing moods at the end of the book. That's Buddy smiling for the camera!

Milepost 4—I'm The Leader of the Pack/Online and Offline

Epilepsy Support Group

In eighth grade I discovered that there was an Epilepsy Support Group for Saint Croix County, one night a month, to talk out troubles coping, fears, frustrations, on job harassment, domestic strife. At first, I was just a member, and then I graduated to 'Leader of the Pack' status. I was leader (co-facilitator) for Saint Croix County's ESG for eight years. And for two years I was contact-person for the WWEC (Western Wisconsin Epilepsy Center).

Gender makeup and number of the group remained fairly consistent—six to eight people, one male and either five or seven females. This didn't prove to be a problem until they began discussing "female plumbing issues." It also gave me an insight into the female psyche that few males could match.

I was leery of writing this MILEPOST, confidentiality wise, but being that it all occurred over 20 years ago, and the situations these women and one man dealt with are important, the way people can help other people in a group atmosphere. I've fictionalized names and combined situations, but let me assure you the circumstances these people went through are real, not fiction.

Agnes "Aggie" A. was in her 70s. She began having seizures in her 30s, after the birth of her first child. She was misdiagnosed as being mentally ill; the child was taken away by the State. She was institutionalized at the State Asylum (as they were called at the time) for 40 years. In a complex-partial seizure, there is a total escape from reality, and the person can easily be misdiagnosed. When she had a grand mal seizure (as they were known at the time), she was "acting up" and she'd be strapped down on a table, tongue paddle in mouth, and given ECST (electro-convulsive-shock-treatments). It was barbaric and brutal but thankfully it came to an end after the following.

The director of the WWEC (Western Wisconsin Epilepsy Center) Luanne Coy was being given a tour of this facility, long since renamed—Wisconsin State Mental Health Facility. An elderly woman handed her a note that read roughly—please help me, I don't belong here. I fall and shake and don't know why. Six months later, after 40 years of misdiagnosed hell, Aggie was free and living on her own in a small, two room house, in River Falls, Wisconsin. Even after years of mistreatment, she had a delightful sense of humor, always upbeat, a truly great lady. It would be nice to think that she was still with us but at the time she would have been in her seventies; that would put her in her nineties now so it is possible she's still alive but not likely. She got beaten up terribly in her grand mal seizures and would attend the meetings with bruises standing out in stark relief from her white skin.

Sally G. was a perky, snippy little gal, preoccupied with a marriage that was quickly falling apart. She was mother of two cute young girls who always accompanied her to the meetings. To describe Sally as hyper would be a severe understatement—today she'd probably be misdiagnosed as having "restless leg syndrome." And no one could explain why, she was on the drug Phenobarbital, yet it had none of the barbiturate's usual side effects—slurred speech, lethargy, drug-induced depression, slowed thought and movement. In some people, phenobarbital has the exact opposite side effect, hyper-activity. She was constantly on the move, clear speech, highly active, she could not put on weight, her mind and body worked like a finely oiled machine. I remember talking to her on the phone about how she'd been up at 3:00 am that morning and been vacuuming the entire house. We recommended she see a different neurologist, but for her, phenobarbital worked, so don't rock the boat, baby.

Depression, she did have, but it was due to her failing marriage and bastard husband. At each meeting, she railed on about him, his inconsistencies, and shortcomings, how she'd opened a savings account in her name and took all the cash that remained in their joint account out and deposited it. There wasn't much left as he'd been buying presents for his little bit of fluff on the side, a 16-year-old blonde, with the morals of a two-dollar-whore. When he found out he was enraged, but she'd already filed divorce paperwork. We all saw her through her divorce and she was an active member until the group fell apart in 1992.

Kelly I. was a high-school-age girl with verbal diarrhea who came to one meeting. Accompanied by her mother, the girl could not keep rein on her constantly yapping mouth. She monopolized the meeting and discussed various activities I'm sure she had no idea about. The way she was cold-shouldered by the other ladies in the group, most of whom were married brought to mind, been there done that or you have absolutely no idea, girl, while she fantasized out loud. Then two jokes that caused her not to be invited back, I only remember one and include this as an example of the low-class, poor taste jokes we sometimes run into—What does an elephant use for a vibrator? Not funny!

Cora, her mother called me the next day to apologize for her daughter's behavior; she'd been scandalized not only at the "potty" humor but the mention of sexual matters. The thing is, it was Kelly who had the seizures—had she had tighter control over her mouth, we'd have welcomed her back; the poor girl definitely needed support of some kind.

Megan L. and husband Dave lived about a mile from our home just outside Hudson, Wisconsin. She was a wood worker, a carpenter, but had failing hearing. Fortunately, at the point I'm about to mention, her hearing was fine.

Doctor Penovich decided to try me on a combination of Fel-batol (felbamate) and Neurontin (gaba-pentin); I'd been in the drug study for the latter when still a patient at MINCEP (Minnesota Comprehensive Epilepsy Program). It didn't work and caused major balance difficulties.

I was in the living room and just like a pine tree felled in the forest, Don went KER-BOOM! The back of my skull collided with the chimney hearth and cut a nasty 3-inch gash. Good thing about having been diagnosed with a thick skull (check out Computerized Diagnostic Testing of the Electrical System, Milepost 2). The one thing I remember was taking a cloth and washing the hearth off so it wouldn't stain blood. It is a funny thing, the memory. I called Meg and she drove over and took a look at the back of my head and said, "We're going to the Emergency Room."

Here I'll introduce a man I'll call Doctor Payne. As I was lying face down on a table in the ER, he cleaned out the wound. I remember he wore gray slacks and white/red pinstripe shirt. He said they weren't going to use Novocain; I should be full of endorphins (natural painkillers) now. It was the first time I had surgical staples without anesthetic and I felt each and every one go in. Sadly this was not the last time I had surgical staples in my 40 year Epilepsy Career. Newsflash to doctors—Just because mentally we aren't quite with it yet does not mean we don't feel pain. We stopped by Taco Bell on the way back to her place; I wasn't hungry. When we got to their place I climbed into a leather-upholstered EZ-Boy Recliner with bath towel under the back of my head and fell asleep, I was exhausted and slept for 5 hours. Meg knew my Dad worked at Oakland Junior High School, called there and left a message. Dad pulled into Meg and Dave's driveway around 5:00 pm and picked me up. We headed home.

A couple weeks later, the staples came out, but it was a breeze. They used what looked like a reverse tweezers to get underneath each and SPROINGed them out.

Meg was a cool lady and I felt really bad when the group fell apart in 1992. She and Sally G. were smaller-sized women and would exchange clothes, as they were the same size. Meg had been on the drug Felbatol for years and was seizure free. Then she reached that particular time in life, she was 45-years-old, when hormones get caught in a hellish whirlwind called menopause, and I received a call from her husband, Dave, as at this point, Meg was nearly stone deaf, and being that she had female problems, I thought a woman Doctor would be just the ticket and recommended my neurologist, Patricia Penovich.

There was a man named Tim S, who also was on the drug Phenobarbital and it had the opposite its usual effect. He was a member of MENSA (a high IQ society) and he didn't really like the idea of being on it as it can have some bad long term effects on intellect, memory, etc. We talked him into a new neurologist, and I believe he switched onto a less side effect AED. I'm not certain though as he and his wife stopped going to the group.

Angie S. lived with Don C., a man from the area in which I'd gone to High School, who'd graduated four years before I did. The first time, they both came to the group together. She only came a few times after, always alone. She had issues she dealt with at work—a canning factory. Angie had tonic-clonic seizures and they insisted she work on the line, where she overheated, BOOM! A seizure would strike her. Of more concern were the exposed blades, knives used to cut out the bad or black parts of string beans. There were far less hazardous jobs, but the supervisor, "High-handed Joe Cool," insisted she work on the line. After a call to the director of the WWEC, and a call from her to the owner of the canning factory, Angie was given a job in a far less hazardous part of the building and a rise in pay. After the change in her employment situation, she stopped coming to the group, maybe venting thoughts and feelings was just not her thing.

Check out the papers for advertisements of Epilepsy Support Groups in your area. If you don't see any call the nearest hospital—The Saint Croix County Epilepsy Support Group met at the HMC (Hudson Medical Center); the workers there will be most helpful. Try the local library—The Star lighter Writing Group met once a month at the Grantsburg Public Library. Open up the Yellow Pages and let your fingers do the walking to the letter E and see if a regional Epilepsy organization is listed—give them a call. Here I have a link that will help you locate your local Epilepsy Foundation, from which you can locate a Support Group in your area. Find Your Local Epilepsy Foundation— you can search by either ZIP code or State http://www.epilepsy.com/

The key word is epilepsy, the seizre condition that approximately two-percent of the World's population share. The secondary, Support—It helps you cope with all the pressures life deals you, frustrations with your living situations or as in the case of Sally G., marital problems, it lets you blow off steam, boosts your self-esteem, self-worth, unquestionably help with your depression, and unless hyped up on phenobarbital like Sally G., usually helps you sleep better. The third word is group, it shows you are not alone, I know how it can feel like that sometimes. The first Support group I attended, I was shocked, literally dumbstruck, there were eight people there just like me. It was enlightening, regardless what other people did, and thought, and said, I was part of a group of "extra-ordinary" people.

There were other members of the group, too, but these were the memorable ones. Feel free to email me—I will respond via email, just when is the question, my email address is strangedetour@grantsburgtelcom.net

High Tech Online Support Group

I started an online support group on the Epilepsy Foundation site—check out the link on the about the author page at the end. So I'm counseling people once again, this time in a high-tech way and I love it; I really like helping out other people, if you have complex-partial seizures or are a caregiver of a person that has CPs, you are more than welcome. Our number is 75, although it is actually 74 as one member, a great guy named Todd K. died of a heart attack in August of 2014. His page is still up, his last post was about three hours before he had his heart attack and died. You can think of the Epilepsy Foundation site as Facebook for people with Epilepsy, their caregivers, I know some neurologists are members and a few psychiatrists—they're the ones who ask; what state of mind were you in after the seizure?

Milepost 5—Surface-Scratched and Beat To Hell (Fashion Model Career in GQ or Playgirl Is Gone Now)

Scars, bumps, bruises

I have many seizure related scars on my body, some visible, some not.

Starting from bottom to top:

Incision scars (reconstructive ankle surgery, steel plate and eight screws)

Four inch on inside of right ankle

Five inch on outside of right ankle

Left knee ACL Reconstruction:

Scar from middle of kneecap seven inches straight down

Lower back:

Two vertical scars:

One on one side of the spine

One on the other

Approximate length(s)—eight inches

Scar diagonally down across back four inches onto left buttock

Upper torso:

Four-inch vertical scar that stops at base of left pectoral muscle (this was from a microphone stand I fell on in a seizure; I think I cracked a rib that time too).

Top of left pectoral muscle/by shoulder joint

Diagonal VNS scar – three inch

Left side of neck – second VNS scar (not even noticeable)

Back of skull:

I've lost track of the number of times I've split the back of my head open (the scalp)

A conservative estimate would be six times

I always wear my hair long in back so that the scars don't show

On the face:

A curved scar just under the left eye, actually right on the edge of the eye socket

I thought it was just a short one-quarter inch scar but closer examination reveals a one-inch scar

When I think just how close I was to being blind in that eye, it makes me furious. I got it in my final stress-induced seizure at the factory I was working at. And the "so-called" normal workers laughed and thought it funny.

Short one-half inch scar high up across the bridge of the nose

One-inch scar further down the nose just above the flare of the nostrils (it's straight and then curved, kind of like a shepherd's hook)

The one that's high up I'll keep as a memento of my own stupidity:

(I attended a Book Club Christmas party, and while there I ate a bar the bottom of which was covered in chocolate. I've had problems with the caffeine connection before. Five minutes later, while I was seated on a sofa, Buddy got real close, hanging his head over my thigh, pressing down hard. I couldn't have moved if I'd wanted to. All his detecting went for naught though. After the party, I was in my apartment, and according to the bloodstains on the mirror I slammed face first into it. The cross-piece on my glasses bit in and while I struggled to regain consciousness, the glasses slid down the nose on the blood that was freely flowing and cut in again, lightly, just above the flare of the nostrils.) I used hydrogen peroxide, anti-biotic cream, and just plain old oxygen to help them heal up.

More facial scars I have no idea about:

Above right eyebrow, halfway up forehead, three-quarter inch horizontal scar, large ugly scar with a big knot of scar tissue

One and one quarter inch scar diagonally close to left temple, above left eyebrow, almost an identical scar to the opposing side, a one-half inch horizontal scar.

More scars on the lower back:

I fell in my apartment, twice, according to the bruises. I landed on top of a floor fan (approximately two and one-half feet square by four inches deep), once on each side of the fan. My entire lower back and the upper half of my butt were deeply bruised and in pretty bad shape. I'm a big guy, just about six-feet-tall, 238 pounds, and I demolished the fan.

Fell again, not sure when, but my back is one big bruise, I'm sure my next door neighbor, Laura, can hear me as I get ready for and into bed, "Ouch! Shoot! Ouch! Shoot!" Well, maybe the words are more choice; I guess I'll have to ask her. Day by day, my posture is becoming more upright without gritting my teeth together and going, "Ouch."

The night before the folks got back from Arizona this year, 2014, I destroyed a floor fan I'd borrowed from them, fell on top of it, but didn't get bruised up this time. Update—the fan still works, the switch on it doesn't; I use it to shift stale air around in the apartment. I plug it in and out to turn it on and off.

My Fashion Model Career is on hiatus:

My epilepsy has pretty much insured I don't make a name for myself as a fashion model in GQ or PLAYGIRL magazine, unless they want the rugged weather-beaten look; at times after a really rough seizure I look like I've been a boxer that went 10 rounds with the Heavyweight Champion—bruises, swollen face, shuttling around like a hermit crab with a limp, often wearing glasses two or three prescriptions too old because I either can't find my current ones or the frames are bent and need to go to the eye doctor to be bent back in shape again.

Currently I'm wearing an old pair of glasses as in the last seizure my apartment swallowed them whole. I have no idea where they are and I haven't been able to find them in the ten days since then. They've ordered another pair at Grantsburg Eye Associates, PA, but they won't arrive for another week or so.

Milepost 6—Experiencing Static Interference on the Radio

On the Job Harassment and the HBU or Psych Ward

THE ULTIMATE DIAGNOSIS IS PARANOID SCHIZOPHRENIA, I TAKE RISPERDAL (RISPERIDONE) TO CONTROL IT, according to a Cousin, Risperidone normalizes brain (psychiatric) chemistry

ALSO IN 2013, AFTER BEING PUT ON BANZEL I WAS ATTEMPTING TO GO OFF OF RISPERIDONE MYSELF, STUPID IDEA, SUFFERED THREE PANIC ATTACKS IN WHICH I THOUGHT I COULDN'T BREATHE, I'D BE WILLING TO DISCUSS EITHER

ACCORDING TO MY MEDICAL CHART, BOTH CONDITIONS ARE ACTIVE, the psychiatric problems are related to the epilepsy, but they are not the cause of the epilepsy; I do not experience psychiatric seizures

I am including this because it actually occurred, none of it is fictionalized, nor are the descriptions of what occurred in the HBU—Human Behavioral Unit embellished at all. The factory I mention is still in existence and employs the disabled and I was grateful for the opportunities offered to me. It provides employment for mentally or cognitively impaired individuals (neither of which is applicable to me) and I am truly thankful for its existence.

The mentally-impaired—I refuse to use the word retarded, as I think it's cruel—are often forgotten in modern day society—at this place they were given a specific job to do, given self-worth, and received a paycheck for their efforts. It was not a Sheltered Workshop, but a recognized work place.

It also employed so-called "normal" individuals, who, during my last year of employment there, created an intensely stressful atmosphere that the administration refused to recognize.

From 1995-2001, I worked in a factory. In 2001, I was under great stress at work and began hearing voices. Doctor Penovich had me come down and undergo testing at Unit 7900—the Neuro Ward at United Hospital—for massive amounts of seizure activity that might cause post-ictal-psychosis. When the brain is bombarded by massive amounts of seizures, it might get a little scrambled; a person might see things not there or hear voices not spoken. There was no such activity detected.

I then spent five days in United Hospital's Human Behavioral Unit—a politically correct term for Psych Ward. It was the most terrifying five days of my life. Carrying my suitcase to my room, I prepared to settle in. One of the Unit's assistants came in. My belongings were searched and piled into have and have-nots. Aerosol Sprays were out—you might inhale and kill yourself. My belt was taken away, shoelaces, sweatpants (the drawstring), anything you might string yourself up with. I didn't hear about thong underwear or bras being contraband; but, as a woman—Nat Lund, in the novel I'm writing says—Elastic is mighty tough. She'd heard of a woman committing suicide with her bra.

At the time I used an Atra razor, it was taken away so I didn't slash my wrists or cut my throat. Five days later I was awfully bristly. I always wear a silver neck chain that was taken away.

Your first night and if you were considered at risk, you spent the night(s) in the suicide room, and continued to do so until it was considered safe for you to join the others. There was one girl who had spent four nights in the suicide room, until she was allowed to join the group therapy session.

That therapy session was like a trip through hell. One never realized how irrational the rational or the depths the human psyche could reach. I write dark fiction, but this was truly scary stuff. Two young girls with dark tans had multiple pink scars on their forearms—they engaged in not too "secret cutting" to escape from the realities of domestic abuse or abuse of another nature, and divorce, a tall African-American man was a schizophrenic, several were suicidal, others just mentally imbalanced, some their parents had sent there as there didn't seem to be any place else for them.

I was on the anti-depressant—Serzone—and spent 20 minutes with Doctor Goering (just like the Nazi General). He said I wasn't depressed; instead, he prescribed the drug—Risperdal (risperidone), a psychotropic or anti-schizophrenic. So, the actual diagnosis is schizophrenia. I hope you realize it takes a lot out of me to write that. On Risperdal, I no longer hear anything out of the norm.

I grew a mental suit of armor working there, the lead workers managed to punch some holes in it with a spate of verbal crowbars, over the 13-year interim my skin has grown so thick I don't need that suit anymore; I'm just saying I can't be hurt like they did to me back then. Age 50 is far from age 37. And, I have my writing to devote my life to.

Dealing with a disability on a daily basis, in addition to the pressures life might deal you definitely puts you at risk for psychiatric or emotional problems. If you are having difficulties, have no fears in confiding in your neurologist. A little chemical assistance is nothing to be embarrassed about.

After a five-day stay in a Psych Ward—my nerves were frazzled and after the almost deathly quiet in the HBU—Human Behavioral Unit—everything seemed amplified. In the HBU even the walls were carpeted in a blue mural that was supposed to appease the mind; all it did was kill any sound. I returned to the IMS—Intensive Monitoring Suite—at Unit 7900 on September 10, 2001.

Milepost 7—Super-Charger under the Hood

The VNS

I returned to Unit 7900, United Hospital, on September 10, 2001. I was told that as long as I was in the hospital, my VNS (Vagal Nerve Stimulator) surgery had been moved up and would occur on the thirteenth. After an uneasy night, try as they might, they could not prevent my hearing the voices of technicians who watched the monitors for their 24-hour video/audio surveillance in the IMS (Intensive Monitoring Suite).

Nearly unable to sleep, I was up at 6:00 a.m., and had breakfast—scrambled eggs, bacon, and Orange Juice—at 7:00 a.m. The date was September 11, 2001. As the morning progressed noise grew louder as a flurry of activity occurred. A black orderly poked his head into my room and said that one of the WTC (World Trade Center) towers was down. I thought this was a sick joke. A nurse came in and punched the button on the remote, powering the TV to on. It was on the History channel. It seemed that all channels had round the clock coverage of the tragedy in which terrorists had taken hold of the heartstrings of every American, and cruelly yanked, ripping them free.

Two days later, Doctor Kirth Davies of Cyberonics, Inc. implanted an NCP (Neuro-Cybernetic-Prosthesis). An NCP is better known as a VNS (Vagal Nerve Stimulator). The VNS is about the size of a pocket-watch—2 inches in diameter, thickness varies with the model number.

The case for the VNS is made of titanium. It houses a radio-active battery and computer controlled electrical—in micro-amperages—generation unit. Two wire-leads run across the upper left pectoral muscle, over the collar-bone and up the side of the neck until even with the larynx (voice box). An incision is made, located in a skin-fold, and the spiral cork-screw-like ends are threaded between the carotid artery and jugular vein and are wrapped around the vagus nerve.

Vagus means wanderer and the term is appropriate as it is the longest nerve in the body—21 inches. It is the root word for vagrant. It is the perfect conduit for sending electrical impulses up into the brain

There are different theories as to how the VNS works. One—the electrical impulse continually fed into the brain makes it think it is in a continual seizure state and chemicals are released to clamp down on seizure activity. The other—that the brain releases a neuro-transmitter that clamps down on seizure activity. I believe my neurologist, Doctor Penovich, believes in the latter theory.

I spent one month at my parents' home on Mud Hen Lake— seizure free. I returned to work at the factory and suffered two stress-induced seizures. It was this, advice from Pastor, therapist, and Doctor Penovich, as well as the hostile, unhealthy work environment that caused me to terminate my employment. In 2002 I decided to become a writer and began going to Starlight Writers meetings once a month. In 2005, I became a member of Northwest Wisconsin Regional Writers, NWRW. Currently, I am a member of WWA, Wisconsin Writers Association. For a year, I was a member of Yarn-spinners, a critique group; they were there when this book was conceived.

A New Super-charger is fitted in

Sometime in June of 2012, I received a call from one of Doc Penovich's nurses; my VNS battery was just about dead and would be dead by the next time a neurologist appointment rolled around. They set up a new VNS surgery for 7-11-2012 for a model 102-R. That morning was the usual lousy Vimpat balance problems but it was so bad by the time they had me seated signing paperwork, a wheelchair was called for. It was an outpatient procedure but I was put fully under general anesthesia, the surgeon was Mary Dunn, a woman who by outward appearances, at least to both my father and I, lifted weights and worked out.

I have one question, why do you have to be naked on an operating table? I can't think of anything with more germs than the human body. But, naked I was under a wrap and blankets of some sort so I didn't freeze to death; it was cold in the operating room. I understand that the cold helps prevent bacteria production.

I was in the recovery room for 45 minutes, much longer than I needed to be according to one nurse. After, I'd regained my equilibrium so I didn't lose my balance when Buddy ran up to greet me, he was so excited to see me he nearly knocked me on my butt; on the way home I ate little more than a milk shake at McDonald's. I had to stay with someone as I'd had general anesthesia so I spent the night with the folks, and returned home about noon the following day. They glued the incision shut so I couldn't take a shower for 72 hours. It took quite a while for the glue to dissolve in the shower or flake off.

Buddy was in fine form in 2012, it wasn't until 2013, the last year of his life that his body began betraying him, getting weaker day by day. Finally, toward the very end, he had trouble controlling his waste disposal—not just once, but numerous times, in the apartment; I just didn't want to admit he couldn't control his pooping anymore.

I have to officially admit that I am a cyborg—cybernetic organism, that is something part machine/part living organism. I have my borg assimilator attached to my vagus nerve and the battery that runs it is radioactive. The Todd K. I previously mentioned had a VNS too and kidded that our piss should glow in the dark.

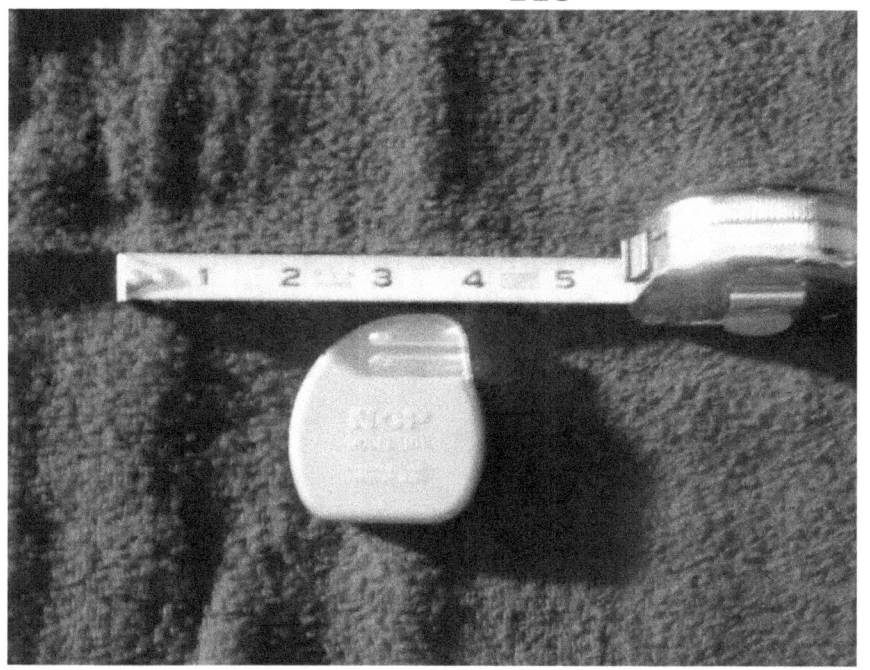

VNS MODEL 101 IN COMPARISON TAPE MEASURE

Milepost 8—On the Watch for Falling Objects

Atonic seizures

My first two seizures were the tonic-clonic type, better known as grand mal. I had been tried on one AED, Tegretol, with no success. I was put on a daily regimen of Dilantin and the tonic-clonic seizures ceased. My seizure type then progressed into absence or petit mal seizures. From petit mal they progressed to complex-partial seizures. At this point, 1977, I had my current neurologist at the time, Noble Jameson; sign out a referral to go to a program sponsored by MINCEP (Minnesota Comprehensive Epilepsy Program).

It was called the 5-Day Outpatient Program. There was a group of eight of us and for an entire week (5 weekdays) we stayed at the Cricket Inn on South East University Avenue, located a block away from MINCEP's headquarters at that time. We were all fitted out in portable EEG units. Wires attached to the scalp trailed behind our backs and were gathered together by loops of elastic. This man-made pigtail trailed down our backs until the wires were plugged into a recording unit that resembled a Walkman. It had a red button that we were supposed to press when we felt a seizure coming on. I have never had a warning, known as an aura, for my seizures. All that week we were not allowed to wash our hair, pretty greasy, smelly, and disgusting. After five days of sponge baths, the feel of a hot shower massaging naked skin and greasy, itchy scalp was like heaven. We were allowed to go out walking through the University of Minnesota Campus. When people asked, we'd kid, "Yeah, the box collects our brain waves." It really was not at all far from the truth. We tried our best to inject some humor into an all too serious subject.

Colin Macgregor, a professor, and his wife were part of the group. Colin had a seizure type I'd never seen nor heard of before. We all hopped in a couple cars one night (some people could drive, Colin's wife, for instance), we went to a shopping mall down by the river, where we didn't shop, as by that point in the week we all looked and smelled pretty disreputable. There was an Indian food restaurant that we went to and I ordered some type of beef that was served raw with burnt outsides like someone had run a blowtorch over it. I was not impressed. I did get some candied fennel seeds that were pretty darn good. We were headed out of the building when all of a sudden we heard a hollow coconut shell sound, and saw that Colin had fallen straight backwards and rapped his skull on the floor. His hand had gone into his trousers pocket and he looked like a baseball player scratching himself. Colin had an Atonic seizure.

We went through NMSQT testing (Neuro-Muscular-Sociological-Quotient-Testing), these tests measured ability to concentrate and focus on task, vocabulary, dexterity, and reflex time. The real purpose of these tests was to determine if we were suffering from toxicity—if we were being over-medicated.

After that week of testing I was taken off the drug, Depakene, and the drug, Mebaral. That was the first time I encountered Doctor "Big John" Gates. The combination of Mebaral (mepho-barbital) and Depakene (valproic acid) had turned me into a virtual zombie. Doctor Gates took me off both, when I was taken off of them, I could think clearly, complete sentences in a normal tone of voice, not a sludgy, slow-motion robot. At the end of that 5-day-period, I became a patient of MINCEP's head neurologist at the time, John Gates, M.D.

Mebaral turned into phenobarbital after being processed by the liver. Phenobarbital, a barbiturate and big-time downer, caused me to suffer depression, lowered self-esteem, all at the tender age of 14. As if growing up with a disability wasn't enough, my first neurologist had effectively cut off my socialization with my peers. Add all the normal hassles that a child going through adolescence had, depression, and lowered self-worth and you've got a lot of emotional baggage for an adolescent's luggage rack. The psyche might not be a car but it too can become scratched and dented.

Superman Seizures

At my last appointment I mentioned to Doc Penovich that I have atonic seizures, she said no, an atonic is a generalized seizure and I have partial seizures, most commonly complex-partial seizures with a focus or origin in my right frontal lobe. I have a partial seizure that mimics or clones an atonic seizure but rather than my thigh and butt muscles giving out and me dropping to the ground, my thigh and butt muscles contract and I'm launched through the air like Superman only to crash land. Being that I was a runner in my youth I have muscular thighs and butt so sometimes I fly quite a ways before landing. So I was mistaken but sure have rapped my hard head a good number of times while being a superhero. These didn't prove to be overly damaging until July 24, 2004.

My service dog—Buddy—and I were out at my parents' home on Mud Hen Lake. I had on relatively new—New Balance running shoes. The folks were seated at the kitchen table and I was standing; Buddy was well out of the way behind me. My brain shifted my body into caped crusader mode and I flew through the air; I landed with a crash, fortunately not on my service dog—Buddy and in the process of landing shattered my right ankle and had what they call a tri-malleolar fracture. There is more to the story and you'll find it in MILEPOST 9—Bodywork.

Milepost 9—Bodywork and Dent Repair

Operations and Body Repair

In 1995, at the age of 32, I was still living with my parents—Grace and Neil. I took a Swan dive into the concrete floor, in a seizure-related fall and busted out my two top front teeth. That called for two crowns that cost $1400 at that time; now of course, it would be much more. That is a sizable chunk of change when you are working in a factory at piece-rate wages. Piece-rate means a penny or so a part, if that. I think I was really getting screwed wage-wise because I could easily turn out 10,000 parts in the brushing division in a day; I'll do the math for you, at a penny a part that comes out to $100 for the day. At the time it was a six-hour day, not an eight-hour day. The highest paycheck I ever received for two weeks work mind you was $374. Two weeks of work entailed 10 days, given 52 weeks in the year, at 5 day weeks: 260 days, that is: $26,000. I may not be a math whiz but something just doesn't calculate there, even after Uncle Sam takes his chunk for taxes, $374 for fourteen days' work doesn't make sense. I never cleared $10,000 (at the time, the poverty level) per year, all my years working; but that is enough of living in the past. I believe my highest yearly wage was $6500.

During my work at the factory, part of it involved lifting 30-40 pound totes with finished parts. This involved a rotational movement. Back in 1999, in my apartment on a Friday night, I fell and as I did so, I heard a "POP," champagne cork noise when my ACL (anterior cruciate ligament) snapped and let loose. If I stepped on a grain of sand or pebble, my left knee would swell up. Gary Kosloski, van driver, had considerable history with Saint Croix Orthopedics, out of Stillwater, Minnesota. He recommended them to me and gave me the name of an orthopedic surgeon—Robert Meisterling, MD. In a consultation/exam with him, he discovered, and here I use a quote, "You've sheared your ACL completely off." In truth, little of the ACL still existed. Surgery was scheduled two days later, at 6:30 am in Woodbury, at their Woodbury "campus."

An icy-cold, gel-like depilatory was applied over the knee joint and partway down the shin. I was given a spinal for anesthetic so as not to interfere with the multiple medications I was on. I was awake for the surgery, something I do not recommend to anyone, if you are given the option of gas, go for it.

I heard every word of the conversation between the surgeon and his team. He cut an incision—about 6 inches long—starting at the middle of the kneecap, down below the kneecap in front of the patellar tendon. A section of this tendon, with bone chips at both ends was removed. I don't know all the intricacies, but two titanium screws, an inch and a half in length were screwed into the thigh and shinbone, securely holding the bone chips in place so that they would graft in place. Doctor Meisterling was less than happy when he saw that the cartilage of my left knee had locked the joint in place. I remember him slamming my leg up and down on the operating table to break it loose.

He then took a tool, like a surgical router, performed a meniscotomy, and removed the sections of "rotten" cartilage, smoothing the cartilage down. After the surgery, I felt no pain, even after the spinal had worn off, but they still gave me two hypos of morphine for pain. They didn't warn me not to eat after and we stopped at Hardees in Stillwater and I took two swigs out of a strawberry shake that promptly headed back up and out. Morphine and food do not mix. There are more details, but two days later, PT (Physical Therapy). They say that PT actually stands for "pain and torture" and I am proof positive. At the start, I could only bend the joint 40 degrees, not bad to start with. I was told in a not-too-gentle-way that I wouldn't be done with therapy until my heel touched my butt.

I don't remember all that the therapy entailed, and I'm glad. They had replaced my ACL, which is of sizable length with a short section of patellar tendon. It was my job to bend that knee almost to the breaking point and stretch that tendon into a new ligament. In other words it was my job to double its length or more; it was agony.

I was downstairs, in my parents' basement in a rocking chair, watching TV. My left foot was behind me and I was gradually stretching that tendon. Then my body shot forward as the tendon reached its full, new length. Up to that point I only had 75 degrees of hard fought for flexion in that knee. After, I had 160 degrees of flexion and that is what my knee is at now.

They tested my knee strength doing squats with various weights and I now have a lifting limit of 50 pounds on that knee. I returned to work at the factory, wearing a heavy-duty black, neoprene brace with metal supports. That, and the promise that from that point on, totes would be lifted for me. They lied. The factory I worked at was funded by one of the major religious organizations, you'd think they'd have valued human beings over monetary profits but no, that wasn't the case; I got shut of that hell-hole in November of 2001. Were I to name that particular organization they have a powerful enough legal arm to quash the book in its tracks; even a self-published book has its boundaries, as for the factory, I'm not going to give that hell-hole free advertising. My supervisor—Max, I do not hold at fault for what happened; it is over and done with, she was a wonderful woman and the only one there that believed me.

In 2004, I experienced a Superman Seizure—sorry, don't know the technical name for them while out at the house of my parents on Mud Hen Lake. I suffered a tri-malleolar fracture of my right ankle. After, I spent a couple days in bed out at the folks; I'd only left the bedroom to attend to biological duties, but my ankle hadn't gotten any better. They took me to the Emergency Room, and at radiology, they X-rayed my ankle and detected a bi-malleolar fracture (fractured on two sides) and fitted me with a fiberglass cast. I was given an option of two Orthopaedics specialty clinics and chose Saint Croix Orthopaedics, the people that did my ACL Surgery. The surgeon was Nicholas Weiss.

There was an appointment at Amery Hospital next; my fiberglass cast was removed, another, more detailed X-ray taken, a tri-malleolar fracture detected. Tri-malleolar meant fractured on both sides and on the bottom. A plaster cast was put on. The ankle was still pretty swollen, so they scheduled surgery for a week later. On that particular day, I remember Pastor David Almlie was there for support. The ankle was still swollen some, but better, so they decided to go ahead with it.

What I mention now has no bearing on what a fine surgeon, nor does it belittle the skills of Doctor Nicholas Weiss. I was given a spinal for the pain of the surgery; unfortunately, they timed it about ten minutes short. I felt every time the needle went in, the thread was pulled through, and as it passed out the opposing side—on the inner side of the leg and the outer. I have a high pain threshold. The bone fragments had begun to knit together, so, as Doctor Weiss put it, "I had to pull it apart and piece it together like a jigsaw puzzle." They used eight screws and a steel plate to hold my ankle together again. The result of all this was that it is body-weight only on my right ankle. I was given a cane and PT assumed I'd be using it for the rest of my life. As of January 12, 2005 I have yet to use it again, unless I've sprained a knee or ankle in a seizure-related fall and need aid for balancing. I had taken Buddy out on January 12, 2005 and forgotten the cane indoors and there it remains. Right now, it is hanging on the clothes rod in my bedroom closet and there it remains until it might prove useful again.

I spent three months—August, September, and October—in the CCC—Continuing Care Center—of Burnett Medical Center, Grantsburg, Wisconsin. I'd like to thank Anita Jensen—a lovely lady, and fellow writer in charge of Social Services for CCC for getting me admitted there. The days I spent there all tend to blend into one another, I did have my recently purchased laptop to keep me busy, visits from friends—(at least to my memory) Kevin, Carol Ann, Doris (who has helped me with Swedish translations for my writing), Pastor Dave, Aunt Betty, my parents, and other relatives, even Buddy, the service dog. He did not like that place at all and I agree heartily with him, nor did he like being separated from me for three months, pretty much only seeing me on the weekends, albeit only for a couple hours per visit.

My last doctor appointment with Doctor Weiss was on November 7, 2004, coincidentally the three year anniversary of my leaving that damn factory; it will be 13-years in nine days.

Milepost 10—There Was a Stoplight at the End of the Tunnel

Goodbye, Vimpat, Hello Banzel

June 6, 2009, Vimpat (lacosamide) was released to the public. It is a complementary drug, to be used along with your other drugs. Before I was taking it, at a conservative estimate, I was having 2 to 4 seizures a week, according to my mother, Grace, 2 to 4 a day. That comes out to 8 to 16 a month or roughly 60 to 120 a month. From June 11, when I started taking it to mid-August, I had 5 seizures. I judge that I've had a seizure by the bruising my body has taken on—back pain, if I'm limping and going by that, my body didn't get beaten up too badly, I might have had dozens of seizures I didn't record as I didn't realize it.

Were I not to have taken it or been able to get it, it would have been 60 to 120 seizures per month as the prior count that had a variance from 8 to 120 per month was with medication, without Vimpat's aid I might have died in status epilepticus. If you are on AEDs and are controlled, that doesn't mean that your Epilepsy has dried up and blown away no matter what the official interpretation might be. Without AEDs, my life would be a car wreck

For a period of time anyway, my seizures were controlled, not seizure free but controlled. Personally, I don't believe there is such a thing as seizure-free, possibly because I've only been so once in my life, while on the study drug—Sabril, and that condition did not last long.

Vimpat was not without its negatives. While I tapered onto it, I had severe balance difficulties. I crawled around on all fours; I crawled to kitchenette, bed, and bathroom. I called it Vimpat drunkenness or "riding the Vimpat tornado." After I took my pills I laid in bed for a couple hours until the dizziness stopped—if you are trying to write a novel, that does not do wonders for your creative output. Finally, in 2013, I had enough of that and got off of Vimpat, September 15 was my last day.

Vimpat, as with other AEDs (Anti-Epilepsy-Drugs), acts upon the brain and in rare cases (1 in 500) there are problems with suicidal thoughts or actions, depression, or compulsive actions. This is true for most other AEDs. My thoughts haven't been depressed or suicidal but at times my thinking has gotten decidedly weird, weirder than usual, anyway.

In 2013, I wasn't being compliant with my meds. This was unintentional; I was having so many seizures I was really disoriented, or 'out of it.' On June 18, 2013 I entered United Hospital's Unit 7900, the Intensive Monitoring Unit, to be taken off of Dilantin and be put on something else to replace it. So, from June 18 to June 29 I was tapered off of Dilantin and tapered onto Banzel (rufinamide). Banzel is great because there haven't been any side effects.

I am currently on 3200 mg of Banzel each day—eight 400 mg tablets, 3000 mg of generic Keppra, and currently—500 mg of generic Lamictal. That is my dosages per day as of 10-21-2014. Banzel is a pricey drug but it in conjunction with the other two AEDs has controlled my seizures very well. It came out in 1998 and after 17 years a drug goes generic; so, in 2015 a generic version of Banzel (rufinamide) will be available; it no longer will be—$9.95 per one 400 mg tablet, yes, that's right—nearly $10 for one pill, in my opinion that's as obscene as some of these pornographic movies and literature they talk about. Even if the generic is half that price it will save my insurance company—Uncle Sam America a lot of money.

Milepost 11—the Owner's Manual

Here is some epilepsy statistics straight out of the E people's toolbox, the Epilepsy Foundation site that currently is Epilepsy.com,

http://epilepsy.com

EPILEPSY STATISTICS:

·Anyone at any age can have a seizure if the brain is sufficiently stressed by injury or disease.

·World Population—approximately 7.2 billion, USA Population—320 million (as of 11-09-2014)

·E people are between 1% and 3% of the World population.

·Males are twice as likely to develop Epilepsy, thus the figure—(Figures are approximated to nearest 100 thousand) For the 1% rate—In the world—total E people—72 million, that comes out to 48 million males, 24 million females. In the United States—2.1 million males, 1.1 million females. For the 2% rate—In the World—total E people—144 million, 96 million males as opposed to 48 million females, in the USA approximately—4.5 million males and 2.1 million females. For the 3% rate—In the World—total E people—216 million, 144 million males and 72 million women. In the USA—6.4 million males and approximately 3.2 million females.

·The Epilepsy Foundation puts the number of new cases at 200,000 every year

·10% of the American population will have a seizure in their lifetime, this is not considered Epilepsy, if it recurs, then the person is diagnosed with Epilepsy

·3% will develop Epilepsy by age 75

·Just to give you some idea of how off base some people can be about E, in this case someone religious; two or three years ago a young woman posted on the Epilepsy Foundation site (check—About the Author at the back of the book for my page's URL, and if you have E or are a caregiver join us, it is like Face-Book for people with Epilepsy). "I could not believe my ears and what happened, about two weeks ago I was attending a tent revival meeting; it was incredibly hot, so much so we were getting ready to leave and head for a movie theater to enjoy the AC there. I had a grand mal/GTC seizure in front of everybody, I think we've all been there at one time or another. I soiled my white dress, major league embarrassment, but what really got to me was when I came out of it, the learned preacher said I had a lunatic demon loose inside and that I must fast and pray to heal me of the "demonic affliction." If you ask me, the preacher was the lunatic and E is nothing to be embarrassed about." I'm holding back this person's name because she was really hurt by the misunderstanding that happened.

·300,000 people have a first convulsion each year

·120,000 of them are under the age of 18

·Between 75,000 and 100,000 of them are under the age of 5

·350,000 African-Americans have Epilepsy, and nearly 24,000 new cases are diagnosed each year—Incidence is greater in African-American and socially disadvantaged populations.

·I'm going to include seniors as a socially disadvantaged group, 300,000 American Senior Citizens have been diagnosed with Epilepsy, the most rapidly growing population group with Epilepsy.

Causes (After effects of):

·Stroke

·Tumor

·Or Cardio-vascular events

TREATMENT IS MORE DIFFICULT, PROBLEMS DUE TO:

·Age related issues

·Use of other medications

·Increased risk of falls, broken bones

·Loss of independence

·Incidence is highest under the age of 2 and over 65

·45,000 children under the age of 15 develop Epilepsy each year. Mine started at age 11, not quite sure what that figure was in 1974

·Trend shows decreased incidence in children; increased incidence in the elderly

·In 70% of new cases, no cause is apparent

·50% of people with new cases of Epilepsy will have generalized onset seizures

·Generalized seizures are more common in children under the age of 10; afterward, more than half of all new cases of Epilepsy will have partial seizures

PREVALENCE

·Prevalence of active Epilepsy (history of the disorder plus a seizure or use of anti-epileptic medicine within the past 5 years) is estimated at almost 3,100,000 in the United States. Note discrepancy above

·Prevalence tends to increase with age

·326,000 school children through age 15 have Epilepsy.

·More than 300,000 persons over the age of 65 have Epilepsy.

·Higher among racial minorities than among Caucasians.

CUMULATIVE INCIDENCE (RISK OF DEVELOPING EPILEPSY):

·By 20 years of age, one percent of the population can be expected to have developed Epilepsy.

·By 75 years of age, 3% of the population can be expected to have been diagnosed with Epilepsy, and 10% will have experienced some type of seizure (not necessarily considered Epilepsy)

EPILEPSY RISK IN SPECIAL RISK POPULATIONS:

(Here I have to state that Epilepsy is a physiological disease, not a psychological, or supernatural aberration (as many, after years of education to the contrary, still consider it).

·25.8% of children with mental retardation

·13% of children with cerebral palsy

·50% of children with both disabilities

·10% of Alzheimer patients

·22% of stroke patients

·8.7% of children of mothers with Epilepsy

·2.4% of children of fathers with Epilepsy

·Men are twice as likely to have E than women, 2:1, but rounded out to the nearest half percentage, women are 3.5 times more likely to parent a child that has E. Pregnancy is something to seriously be considered what with potential birth defects that might be caused by AEDs. I have decided never to father a child, unless my brother gets married, the Miller name ends with me. Two weeks ago I told my parents of my decision; my father was supportive, my mother, a bit hesitant as I'm sure she wanted the Miller name to continue through me, and she wanted more grandchildren, at the age of 79.

·33% of people who have had a single, unprovoked seizure

REMISSION

·70% of people with Epilepsy can be expected to enter re-mission, defined as 5 or more years seizure free on medica-tion. If that happened, it would really be a wild trip. I'd rev my engine and blow my horn if that ever happened.

·35% of people with mental retardation, cerebral palsy, or other neurological condition will enter remission.

·75% of people who are seizure free on medication for 2 to 5 years can be successfully withdrawn from medication (under a Doctor's strict supervision).

·10% of new patients fail to gain control of seizures despite optimal medical management

I'm being honest here; my seizures are controlled to a cer-tain extent, not seizure-free by any means. I spent an hour in an ER this week because my seizures were so uncon-trolled. Banzel has been the cop that wrote the partial-control ticket to my seizing vehicle. People around me know I have Epilepsy because I've told them, I think honesty here with your friends is paramount. Tell them so they won't think you're weird, or high, mentally ill and acting out, though who would want to pretend they have seizures, is beyond my reasoning—and I have met a few in my life, and seeing the pills you ingest—one of those drug abusers you hear about, call the cops or psychiatric people. I'm sorry, but I have no respect for psych ward people, and I do apolo-gize for that attitude. I also realize that they have a job to do and they do it to the best of their abilities. I spent five-days in a Psych Ward once and never plan on spending another second in one.

All the details given, unless otherwise noted came from the Epilepsy Foundation. Details regarding population, World and USA, came from the USA Census Bureau's Population Clocks.

Milepost 12—Empty Gas Tank at the Gas Station

1974

I began having seizures in 1974 at the age of eleven. At that time I was told by my current neurologist at the time—Noble Jameson that the hormonal shift at the beginning of adolescence had tripped the "seizure switch" in my brain to the on position. When adolescence ended, my seizures would stop. I am 51 now and am in the middle of a prolonged adolescence. My first two seizures were of the tonic-clonic type, better known as grand mal. To get a better idea of the mindset or perspective people had at that time, the last Epilepsy "colony" shut down in 1974. That colony existed for one purpose only, to follow the maxim—out of sight, out of mind. I was living under the assumption that he'd died of a heart attack a couple decades ago, but just located his obit in the Minneapolis Star-Tribune; he died of liver cancer in 2007. One sister or brother had died of brain cancer and rather than being an aeronautical engineer, he decided to become a doctor so more people didn't suffer like his family had. He came from the Iron Range, the location all my novels occur at, in fictitious Hickerson County, Wisconsin.

HIGH OCTANE UNLEADED

STANDARD AEDs I'VE BEEN ON

Banzel (rufinamide) In my opinion the best drug I've been on, but a pricey one. It is due to go generic in 2015. Currently one 400 mg tablet costs—$9.95, that's for one of those buggers and I take eight a day; that is roughly $80 per day on Banzel alone. Banzel is doing an excellent job at controlling my seizures. That doesn't mean that I don't have abnormal brainwaves anymore. Vimpat made my balance terrible, Banzel doesn't have that effect at all.

Depakene (valproic acid) The FDA approved the drug Depakene in 1974. Depakene was what I'd loosely term, a "nasty" drug. It was an orange gel cap filled with valproic acid. Lest you think I kid, if the gel cap dissolved in your mouth or on the way down, you'd spend the next five minutes chugging down water to rid it of the horrendous taste and the devastating effects it had on your esophagus. For all its bad points, it really was effective for me, for a short period of time, anyway.

Depakote (sodium valproate) Depakene chemically bonded to a powder state, enteric coated, guaranteed to add fifteen pounds to your weight.

Dilantin (sodium phenytoin) one of the oldest drugs used to treat seizures and one of the most effective, leaches calcium from bones.

Felbatol (Felbamate) caused a-plastic anemia that killed 25 people. I was on it and they took a blood count, my white blood cells began to drop. I was off it in a week; second fastest I've been taken off a drug in my life.

Gabitril (Tiagabine Hydrochloride) not a favorite drug of Doc P's, noted side effect—severe abdominal cramping, like Freddy Kruger jammed his knife-hand into my abdominal muscles.

Keppra (Levetiracetam) One of the newer drugs, been on the market a few years now. Update—Keppra is now in generic form and has been for a few years now.

Lamictal (lamotrigine) Another drug that does its job very effectively, shield or badge-shaped pills, one of the more expensive drugs but worth every dollar. Now available in generic form, in a variety of pill shapes

Mebaral (mepho-barbital) Definitely, it was a barbiturate and I was in a continual zombie-like state while on it. It turns into phenobarbital in the liver, and then it pollutes your bloodstream.

Onfi (clobazam) I didn't even want to mention this one; it was worse than being on phenobarb, I became a zombie and insisted Doc Penovich take me off it after three months. She did, during those three months my writing productivity suffered, I don't recommend it for anyone.

Peganone (ethotoin) is a variant of Dilantin; I was on it for a while, but it didn't work. Always pictured the winged horse, Pegasus, as a guardian angel of sorts when I was on it.

Phenobarbital (Phenobarbital) the granddaddy of seizure drugs. Nearly the oldest used to treat against. The oldest was bromides. Instead of sleeping pills they used to have bromide sleeping powders that were added to water.

Phenytek (extended sodium phenytoin) Timed-release Dilantin. It allows for a continual supply of phenytoin in your bloodstream, no more peaks and valleys

Tegretol (carbamazepine) was the first drug they tried me on, with no success; they put me on it again when I was in my twenties. It makes you photosensitive; I'm a redhead and the only time I ever had a tan was when I was on Tegretol. Noted side effect—diplopia—double vision. Sometimes it was so bad, things weren't just doubled, they were spinning in circles counter to the other.

Vimpat (lacosamide) This was a real bitch of a med that screwed up my balance; I literally had to crawl around on all fours, my knees and hands to navigate around the apartment; Buddy sure gave me some funny looks when I was doing what he was. I even had to crawl into the bathroom, enough visuals. I was finally off it September 15, 2013.

FUEL ADDITIVES

Risperdal is a psychotropic (covered in the MILEPOST titled Static Interference)

Serzone (anti-depressant) It fought depression due to current (at that time) work situation, piece-rate work—slave wages

CELLULOSIC ETHANOL

EXPERIMENTAL "STUDY" DRUGS:

Sabril (vigabatrin) was extremely effective in controlling my seizures, but that control came at too high a price—your vision—hemorrhaging in the capillaries in the back of the eyes, irreversible blindness. Not approved by the FDA

Topamax (topiramate) had been ineffective. Caused incredible decrease in appetite. I lost 25 pounds in 2 months. At the time my stove was still turned on and I thought that a pepperoni pizza tastes like a disc of cardboard covered with ketchup for pizza sauce, grated plastic for mozzarella cheese, and plastic poker chips for pepperoni, and I really like pizza. Known among the diagnosed as Dope-a-max for its ability to cause stupidity. Now on occasion I have a microwave pizza

Neurontin (gaba pentin) Suzie S. of MINCEP said that it only worked in 33% of the cases. That it wasn't a "crystal" drug—whatever that meant.

Zonegran (zonisamide) Caused severe depression and mobility (balance) problems, combined with other medications I was taking. In 1986, I was going to Vo-Tech for a one-year vocational degree in Micro-computer Accounting. We were studying a software program called dBase III, and everything I did connected to it was wrong. Every answer I had in

Accounting 2 was wrong. Mentally, I was in a hole and every move I made, made it deeper. I wasn't suicidal, but was pretty darn close. It also affected my balance. I have a 6-inch scar parallel to my spinal column—lower back—I got when I fell into the sharp corner of a computer desk thanks to zonisamide. I was off of zonisamide in two weeks. I'd chosen office work because it was supposed to be safe and I wouldn't get banged up too bad if something went haywire, if my sparkplugs started misfiring again. I bet you didn't think working on a computer could be dangerous either.

Milepost 13—Driving Rules For the Road

An Overview Of USA Driver Licensing Regulations

Note—this is a condensed version, in alphabetical order. For full details, go online to— http://www.epilepsy.com

Type driver's license or driver's license regulations into the small search bar, upper right hand corner and you'll find a list similar to this. Epilepsy.com is the new Epilepsy Foundation website. All the details came from the Epilepsy Foundation, a great source for Epilepsy education, wellness, support, advocacy, gender related issues, legal support for problems from disability harassment, and many others, just type what you need in that search bar— http://epilepsy.com

If you notice, the period of time for an appeal to a license denial may be relatively short. I believe 5 days is the shortest, Yes, which I take to mean anytime, the longest; get your appeal in as soon as possible. If you meet the qualifications, you deserve to be on the road, the same as Joe or Sally "Normal-Person." For in all honesty, who is normal and who isn't? And, be truthful, it's pointless having a driver license, only to be a bloody smear on the pavement. Some accidents you can walk away from, some you can't, enough said.

For reasons of my own, I will not seek a license, depending on chauffeuring by relatives and friends, it is awkward and not perhaps the best solution, but I believe for everyone's sake, the safest.

Way back when in the 1970s, I went through the classroom training, learning the rules of the road. My father, Neil, was an Industrial Technology—Wood Shop teacher. He also was a Driver's Ed Instructor. The one time we went on the road, I had a seizure and drove the car into the ditch.

Driver's License Regulations Regarding Epilepsy

STATE—ALABAMA

Seizure free period:

6 months, with exceptions

Periodic Medical Updates Required after Licensing:

At discretion of DMV

Doctors required to report Epilepsy:

No

DMV Appeal of license denial:

Within 14 days

STATE—ALASKA

Seizure free period:

6 months

Periodic Medical Updates Required after Licensing:

At discretion of DMV

Doctors required to report Epilepsy:

No

DMV Appeal of license denial:

Within 30 days

STATE—ARIZONA

Seizure free period:

3 months, with exceptions

Periodic Medical Updates Required after Licensing:

At discretion of DMV

Doctors required to report Epilepsy:

No

DMV Appeal of license denial:

Within 15 days

STATE—ARKANSAS

Seizure free period:

1 year

Periodic Medical Updates Required after Licensing:

At discretion of DMV

Doctors required to report Epilepsy:

No

DMV Appeal of license denial:

Yes

STATE—CALIFORNIA

Seizure free period:

3 or 6 months, with exceptions

Periodic Medical Updates Required after Licensing:

At discretion of DMV

Doctors required to report Epilepsy:

Yes

DMV Appeal of license denial:

Yes

STATE—COLORADO

Seizure free period:

No set seizure-free period

Periodic Medical Updates Required after Licensing:

At discretion of DMV

Doctors required to report Epilepsy:

No

DMV Appeal of license denial:

Yes

STATE—CONNECTICUT

Seizure free period:

No set seizure-free period

Periodic Medical Updates Required after Licensing:

At discretion of DMV

Doctors required to report Epilepsy:

No

DMV Appeal of license denial:

Yes

STATE—D.C.

Seizure free period:

Annually until seizure-free for 5 years

Periodic Medical Updates Required after Licensing:

No

Doctors required to report Epilepsy:

No

DMV Appeal of license denial:

Within 5 days

STATE—DELAWARE

Seizure free period:

No set seizure-free period

Periodic Medical Updates Required after Licensing:

Annually

Doctors required to report Epilepsy:

Yes – For loss of consciousness

DMV Appeal of license denial:

Yes

STATE—FLORIDA

Seizure free period:

6 months, with Doctor's recommendation

Periodic Medical Updates Required after Licensing:

At discretion of Medical Advisory Board

Doctors required to report Epilepsy:

No

DMV Appeal of license denial:

Yes

STATE—GEORGIA

Seizure free period:

6 months

Periodic Medical Updates Required after Licensing:

At discretion of Medical Review Board

Doctors required to report Epilepsy:

No

DMV Appeal of license denial:

Within 15 days

STATE—HAWAII

Seizure free period:

6 months, with exceptions

Periodic Medical Updates Required after Licensing:

At discretion of DMV

Doctors required to report Epilepsy:

No

DMV Appeal of license denial:

Within 30 days

STATE—IDAHO

Seizure free period:

No set seizure-free period

Periodic Medical Updates Required after Licensing:

At discretion of DMV

Doctors required to report Epilepsy:

No

DMV Appeal of license denial:

Within 20 days

STATE—ILLINOIS

Seizure free period:

No set seizure-free period

Periodic Medical Updates Required after Licensing:

At discretion of Medical Advisory Board

Doctors required to report Epilepsy:

No

DMV Appeal of license denial:

Within 30 days

STATE—INDIANA

Seizure free period:

6 months, with exceptions

Periodic Medical Updates Required after Licensing:

At discretion of Medical Advisory Board

Doctors required to report Epilepsy:

No

DMV Appeal of license denial:

Yes

STATE—IOWA

Seizure free period:

6 months, with exceptions

Periodic Medical Updates Required after Licensing:

After first 6 months, then at renewal

Doctors required to report Epilepsy:

No

DMV Appeal of license denial:

Within 30 days

STATE—KANSAS

Seizure free period:

6 months, with exceptions

Periodic Medical Updates Required after Licensing:

Annually, until 3 years seizure-free

Doctors required to report Epilepsy:

No

DMV Appeal of license denial:

Within 30 days

STATE—KENTUCKY

Seizure free period:

90 days

Periodic Medical Updates Required after Licensing:

On renewal

Doctors required to report Epilepsy:

No

DMV Appeal of license denial:

Within 15 days

STATE—LOUISIANA

Seizure free period:

6 months, with Doctor's statement

Periodic Medical Updates Required after Licensing:

At discretion of DMV

Doctors required to report Epilepsy:

No

DMV Appeal of license denial:

Yes

STATE—MAINE

Seizure free period:

3 months

Periodic Medical Updates Required after Licensing:

At discretion of DMV

Doctors required to report Epilepsy:

No

DMV Appeal of license denial:

Within 10 days

STATE—MARYLAND

Seizure free period:

3 months, with exceptions

Periodic Medical Updates Required after Licensing:

At discretion of DMV

Doctors required to report Epilepsy:

No

DMV Appeal of license denial:

Yes

STATE—MASSACHUSETTS

Seizure free period:

6 months

Periodic Medical Updates Required after Licensing:

At discretion of DMV

Doctors required to report Epilepsy:

No

DMV Appeal of license denial:

Within 14 days

STATE—MICHIGAN

Seizure free period:

6 months, with exceptions

Periodic Medical Updates Required after Licensing:

At discretion of DMV

Doctors required to report Epilepsy:

No

DMV Appeal of license denial:

Within 14 days

STATE—MINNESOTA

Seizure free period:

6 months, with exceptions

Periodic Medical Updates Required after Licensing:

As frequently as once every 6 months, depending on the circumstances

Doctors required to report Epilepsy:

No

DMV Appeal of license denial:

Yes

STATE—MISSISSIPPI

Seizure free period:

1 year

Periodic Medical Updates Required after Licensing:

At discretion of Medical Advisory Board

Doctors required to report Epilepsy:

No

DMV Appeal of license denial:

Within 10 days

STATE—MISSOURI

Seizure free period:

6 months, with Doctor's recommendation

Periodic Medical Updates Required after Licensing:

At discretion of DMV

Doctors required to report Epilepsy:

No

DMV Appeal of license denial:

No

STATE—MONTANA

Seizure free period:

No set seizure-free period, with Doctor's recommendation

Periodic Medical Updates Required after Licensing:

No

Doctors required to report Epilepsy:

No

DMV Appeal of license denial:

Yes

STATE—NEBRASKA

Seizure free period:

No set seizure-free period

Periodic Medical Updates Required after Licensing:

No

Doctors required to report Epilepsy:

No

DMV Appeal of license denial:

Yes

STATE—NEVADA

Seizure free period:

3 months, with exceptions

Periodic Medical Updates Required after Licensing:

Annually, for 3 years

Doctors required to report Epilepsy:

Yes

DMV Appeal of license denial:

Within 30 days

STATE—NEW HAMPSHIRE

Seizure free period:

1 year, less at discretion of DMV

Periodic Medical Updates Required after Licensing:

No

Doctors required to report Epilepsy:

No

DMV Appeal of license denial:

Yes

STATE—NEW JERSEY

Seizure free period:

1 year, less with recommendation of Neurological Disorder Committee

Periodic Medical Updates Required after Licensing:

Every 6 months, for 2 years, thereafter annually

Doctors required to report Epilepsy:

Yes

DMV Appeal of license denial:

Within 10 days

STATE—NEW MEXICO

Seizure free period:

1 year, less with recommendation of Medical Advisory Board

Periodic Medical Updates Required after Licensing:

At discretion of Medical Advisory Board

Doctors required to report Epilepsy:

No

DMV Appeal of license denial:

Within 20 days

STATE—NEW YORK

Seizure free period:

1 year, with exceptions

Periodic Medical Updates Required after Licensing:

At discretion of DMV

Doctors required to report Epilepsy:

No

DMV Appeal of license denial:

Within 30 days

STATE—NORTH CAROLINA

Seizure free period:

6 to 12 months, with exceptions

Periodic Medical Updates Required after Licensing:

Annually, less at discretion of DMV

Doctors required to report Epilepsy:

No

DMV Appeal of license denial:

Within 10 days

STATE—NORTH DAKOTA

Seizure free period:

6 months; restricted license available after 3 months

Periodic Medical Updates Required after Licensing:

Annually, for at least 3 years

Doctors required to report Epilepsy:

No

DMV Appeal of license denial:

Yes

STATE—OHIO

Seizure free period:

No set seizure-free period

Periodic Medical Updates Required after Licensing:

Every 6 months or 1 year until seizure-free 5 years

Doctors required to report Epilepsy:

No

DMV Appeal of license denial:

Within 30 days

STATE—OKLAHOMA

Seizure free period:

6 months, with exceptions

Periodic Medical Updates Required after Licensing:

At discretion of Public Safety Bureau

Doctors required to report Epilepsy:

No

DMV Appeal of license denial:

Within 30 days

STATE—OREGON

Seizure free period:

3 months, with exceptions

Periodic Medical Updates Required after Licensing:

At discretion of DMV

Doctors required to report Epilepsy:

Yes

DMV Appeal of license denial:

Within 20 days

STATE—PENNSYLVANIA

Seizure free period:

6 months, with exceptions

Periodic Medical Updates Required after Licensing:

At discretion of Medical Advisory Board

Doctors required to report Epilepsy:

Yes

DMV Appeal of license denial:

Yes

STATE—RHODE ISLAND

Seizure free period:

18 months, less at discretion of DMV

Periodic Medical Updates Required after Licensing:

At discretion of DMV

Doctors required to report Epilepsy:

No

DMV Appeal of license denial:

Within 10 days

STATE—SOUTH DAKOTA

Seizure free period:

6-12 months, less with a Doctor's recommendation

Periodic Medical Updates Required after Licensing:

Every 6 months until 1 year seizure-free

Doctors required to report Epilepsy:

No

DMV Appeal of license denial:

Within 30 days

STATE—TENNESSEE

Seizure free period:

6 months, with Doctor's recommendation

Periodic Medical Updates Required after Licensing:

At discretion of Medical Advisory Board

Doctors required to report Epilepsy:

No

DMV Appeal of license denial:

Within 20 days

STATE—TEXAS

Seizure free period:

6 months, with exceptions

Periodic Medical Updates Required after Licensing:

At discretion of Medical Advisory Board

Doctors required to report Epilepsy:

No

DMV Appeal of license denial:

Within 30 days

STATE—UTAH

Seizure free period:

3 months, with exceptions

Periodic Medical Updates Required after Licensing:

At discretion of Medical Advisory Board

Doctors required to report Epilepsy:

No

DMV Appeal of license denial:

Within 10 days

STATE—VERMONT

Seizure free period:

No set seizure-free period

Periodic Medical Updates Required after Licensing:

At discretion of Medical Advisory Board

Doctors required to report Epilepsy:

No

DMV Appeal of license denial:

Within 10 days

STATE—VIRGINIA

Seizure free period:

6 months, with exceptions

Periodic Medical Updates Required after Licensing:

At discretion of Medical Advisory Board

Doctors required to report Epilepsy:

No

DMV Appeal of license denial:

Yes

STATE—WASHINGTON

Seizure free period:

6 months, with exceptions

Periodic Medical Updates Required after Licensing:

At discretion of Medical Advisory Board

Doctors required to report Epilepsy:

No

DMV Appeal of license denial:

Anytime

STATE—WEST VIRGINIA

Seizure free period:

1 year, with exceptions

Periodic Medical Updates Required after Licensing:

At discretion of DMV

Doctors required to report Epilepsy:

No

DMV Appeal of license denial:

Within 10 days

STATE—WISCONSIN

Seizure free period:

3 months, with Doctor's recommendation

Periodic Medical Updates Required after Licensing:

At discretion of Medical Advisory Board

Doctors required to report Epilepsy:

No

DMV Appeal of license denial:

Within 10 days

STATE—WYOMING

Seizure free period:

3 months, with exceptions

Periodic Medical Updates Required after Licensing:

At discretion of Medical Advisory Board

Doctors required to report Epilepsy:

No

DMV Appeal of license denial:

Within 20 days

Again, if you qualify, and can afford it, go for it, go to the website for full details. Just because they say no once, doesn't mean they won't reconsider, the second or third time. The reason I included this MILEPOST is because those 60 or 90 or 180 days, or year can seem like an unreachable goal—it is freedom we all—well, many of us anyway long for.

Milepost 14—Lights That Warn You (A Deer in the Car's Headlights)

SEIZURE-PRECIPITORS

These are the main triggers for seizures; there may be others that people run into but I've run into most of these (except the female only related ones) at one time or another in my 40-year E career.

Male/female changes:

Menstrual cycles

Menopause

Testosterone

Hormonal change

Emotions:

Anger

Stress

Worry

Anxiety

Sleep and wake cycles:

Fatigue

General illness:

Fever

Diarrhea (dehydration)

Vomiting (loss of medication)

Infection

Metabolic conditions:

Low sodium levels

Low blood sugar

Low calcium levels

Reflex seizures:

Flickering lights (photosensitive Epilepsy)

Certain kinds of music

Watching TV

TV screen flicker is more common with European TV as it has a lower flicker frequency

Electronic screen games

Certain thinking tasks (I have this one, although I call it sensory overload)

Eating (Robert, in BACKFIRES)

Heat and hydration:

Overheating—soaking in hot water

Dehydration

Drinking to excess causes mineral salts needed for seizure control to be washed out of the body, those 8 glasses of water a day are not a good idea if you have Epilepsy

Other:

Missed medication (guilty on occasion with this one)

Caffeine (chocolate is a definite no-no, and plain coffee is not a good idea if you have Epilepsy).

Milepost 15—Keep That Damn Vehicle Polished and Primed For Action

A fitness plan:

I've tried going vegetarian, honest, I have—however, you kind of have to actually like vegetables for that to work. I'd eat vegetables and an hour later I was starving and had to eat again to fill up. Sodium—salt is a hidden enemy when it comes to weight loss. Most women are aware that sodium causes water retention; you swell up or bloat and look bigger or fatter than you are. Hate to tell you guys, but it works the same for men.

I know I don't like to, but read labels, calories. Stouffer's has some great TV dinners that are not bad at all for calories—for example, the lasagna—one piece—is only 350 calories, calories from fat—100, fat, total percentage—17%, saturated fat—30%. Stouffer's Roast Turkey is only 270 calories, 80 calories from fat, fat, total percentage—14%, saturated fat—18%. Try to keep your calories at 400 and under each meal.

Eat breakfast, it is amazing the number of people who don't and wonder why they are having seizure problems. A saying you should remember is—breakfast like a King, lunch like a Prince, and supper like a pauper. Eat snacks between meals, carrots, celery, fruit—apples, oranges, and strawberries. This helps keep your blood sugar on even keel and aids you in losing weight.

Something I found out from my brother who once owned a fitness club—Subway Restaurant will make a six-inch sub into a salad—you just tell them if you want lettuce or spinach leaves or both, then you choose your accessories, your salad additions—tomato, pickles, black olives, onions (definitely not my thing), jalapeno peppers or banana peppers or green peppers, I like honey mustard as dressing. There's no bread so it is low in carbohydrates and you tend not to add weight.

One thing about carbohydrates, don't go overboard and cut all your carbohydrates out, we need them for ketosis (the root word for the ketogenic diet)—having an effect on processing glycogen (sugar). Cutting out carbohydrates can cause problems with your seizure control. I learned that from Doc Penovich. Low-carbohydrate diets are a big no-no for people who have Epilepsy. I like to eat, there's no getting around that, but I do read labels now and that alone is a start. Also, I don't buy stuff unless it is on sale. Like any disabled person, I've discovered that money has to stretch for a 30 day-period and things can really get tight at the end of the month. I buy a lot of things at a Dollar Store, and it is worth it.

May I say a word to parents, friends, and spouses? Please let us breathe, we know you love us but for the sake of God, give us room. If we fall and get a bruise, so what, it will go away in time. We can be just as active as (the word I hate) normal people. I know you don't mean to or don't realize it, but love can be stifling. Misdirected protection can become a veritable prison. That said, an exercise program is easier to follow if there are two of you doing it. Don't sabotage your son's/ daughter's/ wife's/ husband's/ mother's/ father's efforts, being healthy and fit is better for seizure control. Don't want your spouse or child walking or biking alone? You'd probably enjoy getting out and spending some quality time together. If you buy two pedometers—one for you, one for them, you can use it to keep track of your steps separately, and eventually, you may both join the 10,000 steps-a-day club. With a 2.5-foot stride, 10,000 steps-a-day comes out to five miles. It is not a contest, enjoy the scenery, the fitter you get the faster you'll walk, the better for your cardiovascular or heart health. Swimming is good cardio exercise, but it is the one activity I do not recommend for people with Epilepsy, nearly drowning twice might be the reason for my bias.

BMI AND FITNESS FREEWARE

There is a website that is free, that I belong to—www.myfitnesspal.com. Join, and support and encourage each other, I'd like to weigh 220 pounds, I'm six-feet tall, at my next neuro appointment—May 5 of 2014. But the best laid plans of mice and men gang aft aglae - oft go awry. Down would be progression in my fitness. It took time to pack the fat on my body and I realize it will take time to get it off again. Well two appointments later—the last appointment was—10-21-2014 and I lost a whole pound. I just made a sizable financial investment in my writing future that after some thought my parents agreed to so trips down to the Country Cafe will have to be cut short, it isn't a New Year resolution—I've broken every one I've ever made but I just won't have the expendable income to go down there except once a week for a Chef's Salad and that alone will take the pounds off combined with a walking regimen. So it's lift Soup Cans, do abdominal exercises, leg and butt exercises, next time Doc P sees me it will visually be a new person. My personality won't change—I'd love to hear from you guys and gals, doctors, even the psychiatric people at strangedetour@grantsburgtelcom.net. I wanted to lose weight when I had Buddy but he was an old guy and couldn't walk far without getting tuckered out. So, kind of in Buddy's memory I'd like to get in good shape again. Next neurologist appointment is 4-07-2015, ten days before my 52nd birthday.

Your BMI (Body Mass Index) is an estimate of your body fat based on height and weight. If you're Internet savvy, Google or Yahoo—Freeware BMI Calculators. There are hundreds. You can also download free calorie calculators, etc. For those of you not of the Computer-age, the formula and calculations are as below:

Weight (kilos) / (height (meters) x height (meters)) = BMI.

1 kilo = 2.2 lb., 1 inch = 2.54 centimeters, 1 meter = 100 centimeters

Jim is 6 feet tall (72 inches), and weighs 185 lb.

72 x 2.54 = 182.88 (183) /100 = 1.83 meters

185 / 2.2 = 84 kilos

84 / (1.83 x 1.83) = 84 / 3.35 (approximately) = BMI—25

There's no getting around the fact that I love to eat, so I'm not going to dictate diet to you. My BMI (Body Mass Index), a ratio of lean body mass to fat is 32.3. Healthy (optimal) BMI is between 18 and 25, so I'm considered obese. Even at 230, it will only be down to 31.2. But, it is a start in the right direction—down. As my cousin Tim says, a pound a week is good, but don't beat yourself up if the number doesn't go down or even goes up slightly.

Don't mope around or get depressed and say, "NOBODY LOVES ME, BECAUSE I'M FAT." If it matters, I love you. Don't scarf down six gallons of Ben and Jerry's or Haagen Daz or drink 3 liters of that healthy Diet pop. Don't order out for pizza—three all meat specials, with double meat and mozzarella cheese, or brown bag a 12-pack of beer and chase it down with shot glasses of whiskey. All of those are extremely fattening. If you want to sabotage your weight-loss goals, you've done so.

I have some recommendations:

Walking, a little further each day, eventually you might work up to the 10,000 steps a day-club. There is a little device that clips onto your belt called a pedometer, and dependent on the model you get, it will count your steps, calculate your mileage (based on stride length), and other functions. You can find them in the Sports section of your local department store. Now that my balance is better on the Banzel, Keppra, and Lamictal combination, I, we are going to begin walking the halls again. I am going to start walking the halls again and here you have it in writing; by my neurologist appointment in October or November of 2015 I plan on being down to 180 pounds and be in far better shape than I am; that will be a 50 pound weight loss—I weigh 230 pounds—but I know I can do it. You can all hold me accountable. I also have that lumpy fat known as cellulite; yes, men can get cellulite too, I have that from my brother who once owned Bodyworks, a fitness club.

Biking—I have a 3-wheeled bike, a recumbent one. Up until recently, I had a recumbent exercise bike, but it was being used more for a clothes-drying stand than for exercise.

Two good brands of Health-conscious food are Smart Ones and Lean Cuisine. I like Chinese, Vietnamese, or Oriental Cooking; other than restaurants I really like InnovAsian Cuisine's General Tso's Chicken, it's a bit spicy, but good and the fat count isn't that bad either. Due to my falling in my seizures we decided it might not be in Don's best interest to use the stove: the open burners and all that; so it is turned off at the circuit breaker and is a stand for my microwave oven now. I only use a microwave, a slow-cooker (crock pot), and a George Forman grill. I also buy food at the local deli.

I'm attaching a chest or pectoral workout, arms workout, and a leg and butt workout, the fitter you look the more fabulous you'll feel. As with any exercise plan, call your neurology clinic and get your neurologist's permission.

Following, I've included workouts for various body-parts. When I mention dumbbells or weight, you can be creative, Chunky Soup Cans have a good heft to them—they are a good replacement weight. You needn't buy the big name brand, the store brand is usually a dollar cheaper and you just want it for lifting purposes. Van De Camps and B & M baked bean cans are about twice the height and weight right around two pounds. So, I call it the Soup Can Plan.

The Soup Can Plan

FOR PECTORAL OR CHEST MUSCLES

An excellent exercise for developing chest muscles, which also will increase bust size, push-ups will build up the pecs or pectoral muscles. On the floor, in a prone or face down position, palms flat on the floor, tighten your upper arm muscles—the biceps and chest muscles, push your upper body up away from the ground. You can add variety and vary which muscles are being developed by changing hand position, fingers straight ahead, fingers pointing back toward your toes, fingers pointed inward from the sides, I'm sure you'll discover others. Build up gradually. Growing up, I could do 50 pushups without breaking a sweat, now I get winded if I do 10.

While laying on your back with arms outstretched to the sides using fairly light weight, lifting your arms, swinging them together until your hands meet over your chest—in a standard flye movement, helps build up chest muscle tissue

Standing, both arms straight, holding a weight in both hands, slowly lifting the weigh up until just above the nipple level, lowering it a few inches, then raising it again will also help build up pectoral muscle tissue.

EXERCISES FOR DEVELOPING THE LEG AND BUTT MUSCLES:

I will list three leg exercises, which in addition to a walking regimen, done with or without weights, will not only tone and define thigh muscles, but will also improve your glutes—gluteal or buttock muscles.

Lunges—standing arms down at your sides step forward as far as is comfortably possible with one leg, opposing leg bent so that knee approaches the floor. The leg you've stepped forward with also is bent at the knee. In doing so you activate the quadriceps (front thigh) muscles, and it is a modified form of squat so that it activates the gluteal muscles (buttock muscles). Hold the position for 3 to 5 seconds; do not bounce as you might injure you muscles. When stepping out of the lunge, drag your heel back; this activates the hamstring (back of thigh) muscles. Repeat on the opposite side and continue for a count starting at 10, building up gradually, 25, 30, up to 50, and more, but only when you feel ready to do so. You can do the same exercise identically with weight. If you don't have dumbbells, that's no problem, you can be creative and use cans of soup.

Here is another one, good for the butt and the hamstrings. It is called a dead lift and it is done without weight, In this one you are standing, raise yourself so you're on the balls of your feet. Don't make it difficult, you can put books or phone books under your heels. Keeping your back perfectly straight, bend forward at the hips, arms hanging down. Lower yourself, still keeping your back straight until your fingertips or knuckles touch the floor, hold for a few seconds, slowly raise up, making certain to keep your back straight, then lower down again slowly, repeat five times, then 10, increasing repetitions slowly. The dead lift can be done with weight, but I advise against it. It is a very familiar exercise for body-builders and competitive weight-lifters.

The Sissy Squat—standing, pretend you're riding an invisible horse. Legs are pretty wide apart, toes pointed out. Slowly lower yourself as if you were going to sit on a chair. Lower your upper body about four inches, you'll feel your quads—quadriceps (frontal thigh muscles) tighten up. As you rise up, do so slowly and tighten your butt muscles, this will work your hams—hamstrings (back of the thigh muscles) and your glutes (gluteal or buttock muscles).

ARMS

Forearms—seated, leaning forward, forearm resting on thigh palm up, while holding onto soup can—curl your hand toward you bending at the wrist. In almost the same position, palm down again curl your hand toward you (back side of hand). This will develop the muscles of the forearm. Build up gradually in number of repetitions; we're not talking the Mister Olympia contest just tight and toned. Wouldn't it be great if your neurologist asked what you'd been doing to keep in shape and you could tell her, "I've been lifting soup cans?"

Biceps and triceps—the upper arm muscles—this can be done seated or standing. Arm straight down at your side, can in hand, palm facing forward. Bend arm at elbow, slowly bring forearm up, can headed toward shoulder, while doing so tighten that particular muscle—it is called the biceps. Slowly lower can and repeat, each time tightening that muscle.

Another biceps exercise—Same position as before, however hand position is slightly different. The top of the can should face forward—the thumb should be on the inner on next to the thigh side. Same motion, gradual, as with the last exercise, however this time you slowly rotate the can in a clockwise direction until palm up and thumb is now on the outer side. This exercise develops the Biceps Brachii.

Triceps muscle—there are dozens, but I'm only going to describe one. The others I think you'll be able to figure out for yourself. Arm position is same as last exercise. Arm is a little out from body. Bend arm slightly at elbow, then straighten it, tighten the muscle on the opposite side of the biceps muscle (back of upper arm). This muscle and the biceps muscle tighten up and tone up easily.

Deltoid muscle—Take your left/right hand and slide it up the arm on the opposite side starting at the wrist, over the forearm over the biceps/triceps muscles, at the top of the arm, shoulder level is a muscle called the deltoid. It is sometimes called the cap muscle of the arm, as that is where it is positioned. Arm position is the same as for the last two exercises. Hanging tightly onto your soup can, keeping arm straight, bend at shoulder slowly raise arm out to your side raising it until slightly above shoulder level. You can both arms at the same time and as you bring them down tighten the muscles of your upper back at the sides, you'll feel them tightening—these are called the lats or latissimus dorsi. You can think of them as kind of a Cobra's hood.

Another delt exercise—arm position same as above. Rather than taking your arm out to the side, bring it forward.

I used to be pretty muscular and had a full weight set with barbell and dumbbells. Bench Presses (basically the same as a pushup, except you are flat on your back and use weight) were dangerous, I tended to overheat, have a seizure, and the weight might crash, possibly breaking ribs or crushing the throat. My Mom got really nervous when it came to me lifting weights, that is nothing compared to Buddy—he doesn't want me to exercise at all and will position his body so he's right in the way. I'd much rather drop a soup can and have it land on a bare toe than have a barbell land on me. The fitness section was written before 2014.

I hope these help you keep your vehicle maintained. Let me know of your successes at— strangedetour@grantsburgtelcom.net. In the subject line, put "soup can." I'm really curious to see what the results will be.

Milepost 16—Backfire Types (Types of Seizures)

EPILEPSY CATEGORIES:

Generalized and Partial (Seizure types I've had and have). This is some shocking information. Epilepsy is just excess static electricity in the brain, sometimes our super-charger gets stuck in the on position it isn't our fault, nor can we stop them by willpower.

Types of generalized seizures:

Generalized—means the excess static electricity within the skull (which is what a seizure is) is occurring throughout the whole brain. It is general, spread out.

Atonic—this is a type of seizure I thought I experienced; please see MILEPOST 8—Watch For Falling Objects. Instead I have what I've nicknamed—Superman Seizures.

Atonic seizures are generalized seizures—and perhaps the most damaging. Also known as drop seizures, your body literally does just that. During an Atonic seizure, a person experiences ataxia or the loss of muscle tone in major muscle groups, the tone in the butt and thighs gives out and the person drops down and back.

Absence—referred to in the past as petit mal, a name that told you nothing, it means "little sick"

Absence refers to a brief absence from consciousness, children often have them, sometimes referred to as "staring spells" and they can be a nightmare to child, parents, and educators.

Picture the following scene. Miss Wiltshire, a 25-year-old, chestnut-haired, 3rd grade teacher has just returned to the classroom from recess with her herd of little learners. Joey Smith has seemed distant, lost in thought all day, and this is what he hears:

"All right class lets open our "seizure" textbook. Everyone turn to CHAPTER "seizure" page "seizure." I want Joey to read aloud to the classmates starting with paragraph "seizure." Those seizures are lapses in consciousness, a little seizure that can drive teachers mad, frustrating child and parents. What textbook does Joey open up, what CHAPTER, what page, what paragraph?

Teachers, unless forewarned by education regarding epilepsy in college or in-services, unless told by parents, given a letter of explanation letter written by Joey's neurologist, epileptologist, or Doctor, most likely will assume Joey isn't paying attention, then possibly that he might have a hearing disorder, a vision problem, or that mentally, Joe just isn't with it.

Joe might then have to mistakenly go to Special Ed, until the teacher there might possibly recognize it as absence Epilepsy. LD (learning disabled) teachers are remarkably intelligent and it is very likely they'll recognize that the "problem" child truly has a physical problem, a disorder that he/she shares with millions of "extra-ordinary" people.

I was mainstream educated, never went to Special Ed, and I came out of it with an advanced vocabulary, a killer ability to spell—I really am a good speller, a high school degree—back in 1981—34 years ago, and a 1-year Associate Degree in Microcomputer Accounting, back in 1987.

Here I will tell you of a discussion I had with a woman from Social Services, who I will call, Mary S. The factory I worked at was, in majority, composed of mentally challenged (or the unpopular term, retarded) individuals, and there were also autistic workers there. The director, James Weiss, decided that all the disabled workers needed to have a Social Worker, myself included. Previous to Mr. Weiss coming on board, the disabled workers were not patronized, not looked down on, and not treated like dogshit. They were considered workers as they received a paycheck just like the so-called normal lead workers who received an hourly wage for their efforts. It was not considered a sheltered workshop; unfortunately, Mr. Weiss saw the World differently. The conversation follows:

"You went to Special Ed, didn't you?" said Mary S.

"No, I was mainstream educated, I have a high school degree, and not a GED either. I also have a one-year-Associate degree."

"No you don't, you're making things up. You went to Special Ed," she was so darn sure of herself, it became extremely irritating.

"You couldn't have because people who have Epilepsy are stupider than "normal" people," said Mary S.

My thought was that "normal" people could be and were more stupid than people with Epilepsy. There is a saying "ignorance is bliss." This does not apply to people who are blatantly ignorant like Mary S. Were it so; I've met many happy people on my 40-year journey on Epilepsy's Electric Highway.

She didn't realize it but she'd stepped on a live wire—me. I wrote a very detailed letter to her supervisor at Social Services detailing the discrepancies (and there were more) and telling them to stay the heck out of my life (although my language was a bit more colorful), and never to contact me again, or I would contact my lawyer. I don't have a lawyer, but have a shirttail relation who is a lawyer who would have sued the pants off of Weiss and Company, and the US Government. Government agency interference avoidance is the way I've maintained my independence for the past 17 years, the number I've lived alone in my own apartment. I now have seniority in the apartment building, meaning I've lived there the longest due to the age of fellow residents and the fact that they keep dying off or moving to nursing homes or assisted living complexes. At age 52 now, I think I still am the youngest resident here at Crexway Court Apartments, in Grantsburg, Wisconsin.

Just imagine that instead of just those four lapses in time, Joey Smith was experiencing hundreds of absence seizures each day. Lets say that each absence seizure is 2 seconds long and he has 450 seizures in one day, that is 900 seconds—15 minutes—of lost time.

As I was explaining, absence Epilepsy can easily be mistaken for mental retardation. Complex-partial Epilepsy, of which a fuller description is given below, can definitely be misdiagnosed as mental illness, or the person being stoned or high on some illegal substance. It is nothing of the kind. Your parents need to be on the lookout for this. Every year, stop by the school and introduce yourself to the principal and nurse, get permission to speak to your son/daughter's teachers (ask your neurologist or Epilepsy Center for some brochures, one outlining your child's condition). This will save your child a lot of pain and embarrassment. It seems there is always one "stick in the mud" teacher and it is your job to educate him/her about Epilepsy, and she/he will be more than happy about it.

Education is the easy part. Tell your child not to expect any special treatment in regard to grades; Epilepsy is not meant to be a crutch for the child to lean on. There's a test at school in mathematics and Joe didn't study but spent the night closeted in his room with his PSP and Tony Hawk. 'Mommy, I don't feel good, I just had a seizure, and I think I should stay home.'

Of course, he's hoping you'll go off to work and he can spend more time skateboarding with Mister Hawk. If he tries that con on you, tell him, all right, get dressed, we're going to the clinic to see Doctor Grumbleby. (Doctor Grumbleby always eats Italian food and his breath smells like garlic.) Don't think your child won't use this wonderful crutch or con, disabled people can be creative in the way they manipulate people.

I worked in a factory for six years and saw the wonderful manipulative machinations of the disabled workers I worked alongside.

I emphasize that I am not talking every person with epilepsy, but it is surprising, the complicated con games some people grow into, without taking into account the consequences on the other party.

If that morning or the night before he had a tonic-clonic seizure and is totally exhausted, which often happens, don't merrily pack him off on the bus. Let him sleep the seizure off. Dave, a member of the New Richmond Epilepsy Support Group, would have a tonic-clonic seizure every time he hopped on the riding mower and got overheated by the sun. (Some people are slow-learners). Dave had to sleep for an entire week after. No two seizures are ever alike, just like no two fingerprints are alike; they might be similar and might look the same to some casual onlooker. But they are all different, even in some minor way.

Tonic-clonic—also a generalized seizure, what I call "Hollywood Grandstand" seizures as the GTC (generalized-tonic-clonic) or grand mal seizures are what most people think of when they hear about epilepsy, if they consider us at all that is. GTC was referred to in the past as grand mal, again a no-name meaning "big sick"

The name refers to muscle tone—tonic—loss of natural muscle tone, muscles contract to the point that all natural features are lost. And clonic—refers to the tightening and loosening aspect. The action "clones" itself or repeats itself. What looks like shaking is actually frenzied tightening and loosening, contracting and relaxing of muscles all over the body at the same time as abnormal electrical signals are being sent to control centers all over the brain. Afterward, as in Dave's case, the person is utterly exhausted. It's like he has been weight lifting with all his muscles at the same time. I have another experience to relate about tonic-clonic seizures. At the time I had never seen another seizure in my life—let alone one so active and vocal as a tonic-clonic seizure. Other than those two of Mister Stohr's I witnessed in 1979, that is.

I was a patient at MINCEP at the time. My neurologist was "Big John" Gates, an imposing man, strongly built, with a bushy black beard. I was admitted to the Neurology Ward at the University of Minnesota Hospital. This was my first stay in an IMS (Intensive Monitoring Suite) with 24-hour video and audio surveillance. It was a two-bed room. My roommate was named Robert. Robert was severely mentally-impaired, although at the time, the medical personnel used the term retarded, but really enjoyed doing jigsaw puzzles, and he was quite good at them. No one told me he had grand mal—as they were called at the time—seizures. What happened was totally unexpected.

We'd had breakfast at about 8 am. Robert then put on his helmet, they used either football helmets or in my case, an XL hockey helmet (not only is my head documented as being hard, but it is also exceptionally large—so I'm big-headed, hard-headed, and bull-headed—incredibly stubborn at times), origins unknown. He was sitting in a chair nearly in the middle of the room. In front of him was a four-foot by five-foot board with a large-pieced jigsaw puzzle on it. It had been 45 minutes since we ate, you could have set your watch by it. I heard a sound that curdled my blood. When a tonic-clonic seizure starts, the muscles of the diaphragm tighten and air is forced high-speed through the vocal chords—this, I learned later is known as the epileptic shriek or cry. It sounded like the cry of a huge predatory bird—possibly a super-sized eagle—but it was worse than that. It was like the sound created when someone scrapes fingernails across a blackboard—a noise that drives me up the wall. The puzzle board went flying; pieces went to every corner of the room. EEG technicians and nurses hurried in to administer first-aid, what there was basically to turn him on his side so fluid drained out of his mouth after his convulsions ended, oh, he vomited up his breakfast. Another step was to loosen any clothing around the neck so he could breathe, but he was still in his "jammies" so they didn't need to, and to remove any objects in the way, so he didn't get hurt by striking them.

They got him roused and he wanted a snack—I think they brought him applesauce. I'd totally lost my appetite. Forty-five minutes later, a repeat performance, flying puzzle board included. It happened six times that morning. Like the aforementioned Dave, the EEG people were slow learners—they didn't recognize the connection between his eating and then his seizing. On the fourth, he was seated in the chair and undid the strap on his helmet and took it off, I tried to talk to him, but he was deaf to the world. I knew he was like a rocket on the launching pad ready to blast-off or explode. I saw his body tighten up, he stood up in his chair, then, dropped forward, slamming his unprotected forehead into the puzzle board that had no give. This time instead of the puzzle board flying, blood did. I vocalized loudly and screamed for help and "Big John" Gates rushed into the room. He grabbed hold of Robert's legs and pulled him, half flying to the floor where it was free of obstructions—where he wouldn't hurt himself. I don't remember much else that happened as my heart was beating at 160 bpm (beats per minutes). This time Robert had stitches put in and either "Big John" Gates put them in or another Doctor did. He had two more tonic clonics—same scenario—and my nerves were shot. I'd never realized how loud, how violent a tonic clonic seizure could be. They called Robert's parents in Pittsburgh, Pennsylvania and told them, sorry, but there was nothing they could do for Robert, and the next day, I got a new roommate.

I'll call the man Tim Finglegruber, he'd just had a partial corpus callosotomy and for a time anyway was seizure-free. I saw him several years later, at least I think it was him and he'd had a full corpus callosotomy performed on him. This particular person was in a wheelchair, but as an effect of the surgery or high medication, he was totally unresponsive. I tried shaking hands with him but no response to my hand gesture at all. The corpus callosum is a fibrous band of tissue that connects the two hemispheres, or halves, right and left of the brain. In a corpus callosotomy, that band is cut either partially lengthwise, or fully, the entire length with the hoped effect of preventing the excess electrical charge from passing from one hemisphere to the other. Partial Seizures:

(There are many types but I've only experienced two)

Complex-partial (also known as temporal lobe Epilepsy or at one time psychomotor)

I have my Superman Seizures, and fly through the air like the Man of Steel only to crash land, often getting bruised bad and should I hit a wall, caving in the sheetrock (gypsum board). The administration here at Crexway Court know all about my seizures because I've told them and on several occasions Leo, the custodian, has given me a ride up to the ER for a short stay to have the back of my scalp stapled together again.

Buddy and I were out at my parents, at their house on Mud Hen Lake. I'd recently gotten new leather New Balance running shoes. I was standing in the kitchen, talking to my parents, who sat at the kitchen table; I had a Superman seizure, my thigh and butt muscles contracted and I was launched into the air; I landed in such a way that I fractured my right ankle badly—a tri-malleolar fracture that caused me to have reconstructive ankle surgery, eight screws and a steel plate. I go into a more detailed explanation in MILEPOST 9—Bodywork.

I learned at my next neurologist appointment, that Dilantin would leach the Calcium out of your bones. I've been on Dilantin for almost 40 years now or it's extended release version Phenytek. I now take Calcium with Vitamin D, and a daily multi-vitamin. Before taking any new substance, for instance—minerals or vitamins call your neurologist and get her approval.

Noble Jameson, my first neurologist, used the term TLE—temporal lobe epilepsy—as seizure type for my complex-partial seizures. Simply put, the name means complex—for complex movement and partial—involving one part of the brain. Originally, the focus, or starting point for my seizures was thought to be the temporal lobe. I learned just recently, about 3-years-ago, that the focus actually lies in the right frontal lobe; so, I have FLE—frontal lobe epilepsy, but complex-partial seizures. At an Epilepsy Symposium or series of lectures, one speaker said that anything, anything you can do normally, you can do abnormally in a seizure. That statement is pretty broad and vague to me.

Complex-partial seizures might involve random move-ment—for instance, I've been holding pencils or pens in my hand and either dropped them in a seizure or been unable to prevent myself from snapping them in half. Possibly, I might grasp my legs, grab hold of my watch band and twirl it round and round on my wrist, I've unlocked car doors in moving vehicles which is why I have always, even when it wasn't the in thing, worn a seat-belt. I might stand up and walk, which was of some concern as I live on the second floor of an apartment building on the end, right next to a staircase. Fortunately, there are two doors in between and that alone is enough to turn me around and send me walk-ing in another direction. You might say it is like a sleep-walker, only with amplified confusion of thought in my mind. It is easy to see how, in the case of Aggie A., it might be considered to be mental illness.

Milepost 17— What to Ask Your Mechanic If Your Engine Idles Roughly

Your brain is like the engine in a car—it controls what we do and where we go—and some of us have faulty electrical systems. We have an onboard computer that controls what we think, feel, and remember. It is your and your neurologist's job to make that engine run as smoothly as possible, the woman I have to take care of my engine is a mechanic without an equal. Thank you Doc Penovich—Patricia E. Penovich, M.D.

QUESTIONS FOR THE MECHANIC - THE DOCTOR

1. Would you please let me know what my fluid levels (drug levels) are by phone, email, or snail mail?

2. Do you think I'd be a candidate for an engine overhaul (neuro-surgery)? I've heard that sometimes an engine runs smoother with fewer parts in the way.

3. Could I be fitted with a turbocharger (VNS)? I understand it may help my engine run smoothly.

4. Are there any experimental fuels (drug studies) I might qualify for?

5. Would it be possible to go with just one fuel (drug monotherapy) or will best control be achieved through a mixture of fuels?

6. (For females:) Do you think my monthly cycle or menopause or spastic adolescence hormones have an effect on my seizure control?

7. (For both males and females:) Will any of my AEDs have an effect on my sexual performance?

8. (For both males and females :) Can I participate in activities and sports?

9. (For both males and females :) What do I do if they laugh and make fun of me? My own answer would be to laugh right with them—it takes the fun out of harassing someone, when you aren't visibly affected. It is going to hurt a lot, and realize that just having Epilepsy has made you a stronger person. Think, they have absolutely no idea of what reality is all about, but I do. I live with reality every day, but I deal with it if it happens. I'm not going to let you dictate how I run my life—you aren't going to ruin my life.

·Your reflexes will be tested and each reflex given a number.

·Your balance will be tested to see if all your parts are in alignment

·You may be given a memory test to check out the data-holding capacity of your onboard computer.

·You might have an EEG (electroencephalogram), wire leads will be attached to the hood to detect abnormal electricity—faulty circuitry.

·The technician will check to see if there is any jitter in your windshield wipers at their outermost edge (check for nystagmus).

·If you have a VNS (vagal nerve stimulator), your turbocharger will be given a diagnostic—current will be run through it to check on the power level in your battery and it will be tweaked by an expert technician, your neurologist or epileptologist, so that it is running at optimal efficiency.

Milepost 18—An Engine Overhaul Doesn't Mean You Win The Race

I know five people who have had neuro-surgery—an engine overhaul—who've had pieces removed from their engine—brain—that were thrown away, held as bad or useless anymore. One is seizure free.

Most people say isn't that great, one out of five, that's 20%, that's damn good odds, I'd say. Given that the average efficacy of any given AED is 33%, not bad at all. However, people, the true numbers are much darker than that. Out of those people—four women, one man, they had 12 neuro-surgeries; that comes out to 8.333 percent. If my odds were that crappy I'd never go to the casino again, unless to the seafood buffet.

They never talk about the physical and mental deficits you'll have afterward or the amount of physical and occupational therapy you'll have to go through, and there is no guarantee that you'll be seizure free after, one out of 12, pretty crappy odds.

One woman, after three TLCs (temporal lobe corrections or lobectomies) had so much bad brain removed now she only has a fourth grade reading level.

The man, who had a heart attack last August and died, had three TLCs, and yet still his seizures were uncontrolled and he had to be fired from working at a major grocery store chain out East somewhere.

One woman who isn't fond of the type of fiction I write has a brain that no longer recognizes she has a right leg. She spends much of her time in a wheelchair now because she feels safer there in case she should have a seizure.

One woman, a true Southern Belle has had four TLCs and is still uncontrolled.

The seizure free one, she was a voluntary first reader for this memoir, The Lightning Storm Within: Reflections in the Rear-view Mirror, she's still in her 20s and her young age may have been a helping factor in her recovery. She had to go through a load of therapy, physical and occupational, after.

They never tell you that 4% of the people that have the surgery never even make it off the table to tell the tale.

Milepost 19—Why Does E Freak People Out?

I am a member of the Epilepsy Foundation's NING Social Network and I started a discussion in one of the groups I belong to. I wanted lots of comments so I titled the discussion—Why is Epilepsy Freaky? (a reference to other people's attitudes toward the E people). Think of it as Facebook for people with Epilepsy. If you join, my user-name is Don Miller, go to my page and you can read all the replies to the discussion. Check in the back in About the Author for my page URL, please join, all E people, family, and caregivers are welcome. We actually have a few doctors, and psychiatrists; they're the ones who ask, 'What state of mind were you in after the seizure happened?' I thought people might want to hear from people who actually have epilepsy. Send me a friend-request, I won't turn you down. I have friends from around the World, one gentleman, and a fellow writer lives in the United Kingdom.

Can anyone tell me why the word epilepsy freaks people out? It's like we're lepers and they don't want to catch the dread disease. It is not epileprosy that we have. Epilepsy is not contagious, people. Hylephobia means fear of Epilepsy.

1. Plain and simple—Ignorance is bliss. It's up to us to educate others.

2. When I was growing up, people associated Epilepsy directly with mental retardation (my little brother is both)

and unfortunately, the stigma of the facial features persists. I'm Epileptic, but not mentally retarded and I do not have features consistent with either of my siblings, and some people assume I caught it from my little brother. Yeah, I know it sounds dumb. Not to let my age show, but my brother's first seizure occurred when I was nine and he was six, while we were in quarantine with our mother because my brother had 2 different types of measles and chicken pox all at once. At the time, they quarantined anyone with German measles. I've stopped telling people that part because it gives the misconception that I caught it from my brother. I just try to explain what I learned back in the early 70s; it's an electric short of sorts, then I give people the look of duh...didn't you know. I think people would rather believe it's some kind of disfiguring disease, otherwise how else could you tell someone has Epilepsy. OMG, they can look and act normal. P.S. Most of the people I come in contact with have never even heard of Epilepsy...sad isn't it.

3. It is up to us to educate, but it's sad because they didn't pay attention in health class in school. My niece, who is in 7th grade said in her health book it does have something about it in there, not a lot, but enough to know a little something

4. It's very true. Lack of education on it. I've run into so many people who simply don't know or understand what E is. It truly is up to us to educate as very few people out there will do it for us. Some people think it's caused by drugs, or again, a mental issue, not a neurological issue. People simp-

ly don't understand it, some don't want to, and often what people don't understand scares them. That's why I believe advocacy and awareness are so important. All we can really do is get the word out.

5. But I will say, I am with you on this one. Why Epilepsy, of all things, I don't entirely understand. I have thought about this many times. I believe it's a combination of all the things mentioned, as well as the silence of those living with E. Ultimately, the "whys" aren't so important. It's a matter of what we're going to do about it. We can either wait for someone else to do something, which we just can't count on happening, or we can make a difference ourselves!

6. I may be wrong, I hope so. I think people who don't understand and know what Epilepsy is think we are not able to function in life. Since there is something that is wrong with the brain. They think the BRAIN, they are deformed, slow. They think we look different...I had a lady walk up to me at a Health Fair. She said, "Do you have Epilepsy? You don't look like you do!" I was so mad. I had to bite my tongue. I wanted to say, "What am I supposed to look like?"

7. Why do people think that epilepsy is freaky? Well, could they be uneducated bout it? At my last job I told my supervisors that I do have petit-mal seizures, epilepsy and even though I am on several different meds. I still may have a seizure. Well, within one month I had three at work. After the last one, I came back with a doctor's note in my hand, gave it to my supervisor, she and the store manager along with

my job coach, spoke to some person at the major office and they let me go. I still can't believe it. I looked at the doctor's note and he had some things checked off on there that he says that I can't do. One of those things is climbing a ladder. I thought, hell I do that at home all the time with no problem. But, it suddenly came to me that it is a money issue. They know that I do a great job all the time, and if I needed help to get something down I would ask for it. I was a greeter. And a great one. A lot of customers will miss me and I will miss them. Oh well, I am sure you are tired of reading my story. God Bless

8. I have Epilepsy from an accident when I fell out of my high chair as an infant. My eyes rolled back into my head, my parents freak out, and took me to an emergency room. 11 years later, my seizures began. I had never heard of epilepsy or seizures until then. 32 years later I am still on medication, still have seizures, but the difference is I wake up every day thanking God that I am alive. I read my WORD and I think God keeps me alive for a certain purpose. Maybe my seizures are just a thorn in my side and I should not complain? God Bless.

9. The fear of the unknown. As stated before ignorance is bliss. Just like if an ambulance stops at your neighbor's house. All have to stare and wonder. Yet not do a thing, unless they have some sort of a medical background or some sort of knowledge base

Milepost 20—Collector Vehicles on the Showroom Floor

FAMOUS E PEOPLE

Please realize that this is only a partial list of famous E people.

Agatha Christie: the prolific novelist, her PR people say she had psychic fugue states. The description of them sounds a lot like a complex-partial seizure to me.

Alan Faneca: An American Football Guard, seizures started at age 15, takes carbamazepine (Tegretol) that controls his E

Alexander the Great: Greek King

Alfred Nobel: inventor

Alfred the Great: Anglo-Saxon King

Aristotle: philosopher

Bud Abbott: producer, actor, director, comedian (Abbott and Costello)

Charles Dickens: writer

Danny Glover: actor, had epilepsy in his youth but outgrew it, something my first neurologist—Noble Jameson told me I would do; it didn't happen

Edgar Allan Poe: author

Edward Lear: artist, illustrator, and writer

Florence Griffith-Joyner: Flo-Jo, dubbed by the press "the fastest woman in the world," gold medalist Olympic track athlete. Suffocated and died in a nocturnal seizure in 1998

Fyodor Mikhailovich Dostoyevsky: writer

George Frederick Handel: composer

Hal Lanier: pro baseball player and manager, developed E after a severe beaning

Hannibal: military commander and tactician

Hector Berlioz: composer

Hugo Weaving: actor, (Elrond in The Lord of the Ring trilogy and The Hobbit; The Matrix, as the head bad guy). Hugo has been seizure free for 18 years now.

Jerry Kill: head Coach of the University of Minnesota Golden Gophers football team

Jimmy Reed: his diagnosis of E was delayed because they thought it was delirium tremens

Julius Caesar: Roman Emperor, had what at the time they called "the falling sickness"

Leonardo Da Vinci: architect, botanist, musician, scientist, mathematician, engineer, inventor, anatomist, painter (The Mona Lisa and the Last Supper of Jesus Christ), sculptor, and writer.

Lewis Carrol: author

Lindsey Buckingham: guitarist and lead singer for Fleetwood Mac

Margaux Hemingway: model, actress, sister of Mariel Hemingway, granddaughter of writer Ernest Hemingway

Martin Luther: monk, founder of the Lutheran Church

Michelangelo: sculptor

Napoleon Bonaparte: leader of France, general, may have had E all his life

Neil Young: musician, composer, treats E holistically, that might mean a little herbal help

Nicolo Paganini: violinist, violist, guitarist, and composer

Peter Tchaikovsky: composer

Prince John: British Prince, locked away from public view, to prevent shame on the House of Windsor; there is nothing shameful about E you Royal people

Pythagoras: philosopher, mathematician

Richard Burton: actor, had many medical problems, chiefly among them: alcoholism

Sir Isaac Newton scientist

Theodore Roosevelt: soldier, historian, explorer, naturalist, author, politician

Tom Smith: Former Scottish International and Northhamptom Saints rugby player has had E since 18, seizures only occur at night (nocturnal seizures)

Truman Capote: writer

Vincent Van Gogh: artist

That's 36 men and three women.

Milepost 21—And Hopefully Not a Ride on Dead End Street (SUDEP) Sudden Death in Epilepsy & Suicide

SUDEP

People who continue to have seizures are at greater risk for SUDEP which is why preventing seizures and other problems is so important. The most serious complications are injuries and of course dying from your epilepsy. This section gives information on one of the most common ways of dying from seizures: Sudden Unexpected Death in Epilepsy which is abbreviated SUDEP.

WHAT IS SUDEP?

SUDEP is the sudden unexpected death in someone who has epilepsy who was otherwise healthy. No other cause of death is found when an autopsy is done. Each year more than 1 in every 1000 with epilepsy people die from SUDEP. If seizures are uncontrolled the risk of dying from SUDEP increases to 1 in 150. These sudden deaths are rare in children but are the leading cause of death among young adults with uncontrolled seizures.

WHAT HAPPENS?

The person with epilepsy is often found dead in bed and doesn't appear to have had a convulsive seizure; about a third of them do show signs of a seizure close to the time of death. They are often found face down; no one is sure of the cause of death in SUDEP. Some researchers think that a seizure causes an irregular heart rhythm. More recent studies have suggested that the person may suffocate due to impaired breathing; fluid in the lungs; and being face down on the bedding.

CAN SUDEP BE PREVENTED?

Until further answers are available, the best way to prevent SUDEP is to lower your risk by controlling seizures.

Paying attention to managing your seizure medications as best as possible, taking them regularly and preventing seizure emergencies is all part of this.

SUICIDE

Two studies on suicide in epilepsy have found a higher risk of death from suicide in people with epilepsy, ranging from 3.5 to 5.8 times higher than in the general population. Suicidal ideation or thoughts of suicide are also a problem for some people with epilepsy with past or current problems with mood disorders. Suicidal thoughts and mood disorders may contribute to risks of death in people with epilepsy.

Many thanks to the Epilepsy Foundation for the above information.

Milepost 22—Slippery when Wet

A SEX-QUESTIONNAIRE

I decided not to include this Zen of Epilepsy Life Lesson in the original epilepsy memoir I wrote, but this one is different and if you ask any of my writing friends, Don Miller is more than a little crazy or Fellow writers say that there's madness in Don's method, I point out that madness is mine alone and no one else's. Not my unofficial mentor: Stephen E King, my good writing friend who I sent a large-print version of the original epilepsy memoir I self-published in 2014, in time for my 51st birthday and Olivia Hussey's birthday on 4-17, it was Olivia's 63rd birthday. Steve hasn't contacted me though he surely will, being a fellow writer. He has my address; my landline #; my cell #; and my strangedetour@grantsburgtelcom.net email address. Come to that I no longer have the cell so that number is pretty much useless the title of that book is Detour: A 40-Year Epilepsy Memoir. I also included in the shipment to him, an RP Detour: A 40-Year Epilepsy Memoir for his daughter who is a minister of some sort.

Masturbation

Not usually considered a big deal any more, but divided opinions persist. It is obviously not an expression of love between two people, and in that way it is deficient as an expression of love, but it also does no harm to another. So, in that way, it does no evil, unless the harm is in some way to one's self. I wrote the following for a Northwest Wisconsin Regional Writers topic assignment, I had to change our ages and the woman's name, places names, created the humble county of Jefferson in the state of Wisconsin. The topic is "mailbox" and I decided to approach it from a musical lyric angle...

It's in the eye of the beholder or what you're beholding or doing while you're beholding yourself Cherry

So, Cherry, masturbation isn't looked at the bad way it used to be by the Jesus Saves all... You were wrong in your assumption about it. But just what had Mom said when she caught you? If you want my honest opinion, I don't see anything more wrong with masturbation than French-kissing. I really loved to French kiss, Cherry had a problem with it, what she did not have a problem with the solo-sex long after we broke up and according to our conversation, since she was naked and six and discovered touching a certain part of her created pleasant feelings. I'm not going to be judgmental, I've spent much too much of my own life being judged, does it bother me that she masturbates or masturbated while we were going steady together, and according to our conversation since 1984 and she was a senior in high school? No, if occasionally an orgasm, even a masturbation orgasm makes her feel good, more power to you Cherry. Now she lives in some group home in Edgerton, Hickerson

County. I'm assuming that masturbation or being caught masturbating is not grounds for eviction.

Masturbation is not what you'd call party conversation; there is still a stigma about epilepsy, despite years of teaching to the contrary. There is a stigma about masturbation or masturbating, jacking off, jilling off, turning on, the big O, and other nicknames. I'm giving you my honest opinion here, I don't think there's much to get uptight about or as Slick Willie J, "it is deficient as an expression of love, but it also does no harm to another. So, in that way, it does no evil, unless the harm is in some way to one's self." Views about E have changed over time, and perhaps views about masturbation will change over time too. I sure hope Cherry is happy no matter what venue she uses for sexual expression.

Do I think masturbation is wrong or evil; I share the opinion of the Jesus Saves All Church of the Muddy Waters, at least Reverend William Johnson. Cherry apparently had no problems with physically self-loving herself and if our conversation was right, did it often and frequent enough to be caught by her mother.

I've lived 18 years, possibly 19 years by the time this is published independently and haven't had a girlfriend since 1992, due to the horrendous potential birth defects caused by anti-epilepsy-drugs I've decided to be celibate, not to have sex with a woman or man, even protected sex, when Cherry and I split up, it was a simple mathematical equation: $1 + 1 = 2 / 2 = 1$. 1 stays in Hickerson County and 1 eventually goes from Stillwater, Minnesota; Hammond, Wisconsin; Hudson, Wisconsin; Somerset, Wisconsin; and Grantsburg, Wisconsin. When we were still together and making out, not having sexual intercourse she introduced me to what is known as slow-dancing, swaying to the music, me and my girl. Apparently sometime during our relationship she began dancing to the one person tango, and after the split, we no longer were mutually amicable. Now we hadn't seen each other or for that matter, French-kissed and she had the audacity to say, "I bet you jack off all the time just like I masturbate or get myself off as often as I can and I'm not going to stop because it feels too damn good," being that I hadn't seen her in a decade and a half, whether or not was not information she deserved to know. I will tell you honestly that I didn't answer her on that one. I honestly did love her, you know, and cared for her but she wouldn't give up the bottle and I have no place in my life for drunkards. I feel free to divulge our rocky relationship because I give no names or place names; I stole the name Hickerson from Joel A. Hickerson, a grave in our local Riverside Cemetery. I write what I loosely term "dark fiction fantasy" and characters do have sex, and frequently masturbate to the consternation of parents, I've taken a vow never to have sex with a woman. At the end of the book, in the bibliography, I mention a book by a woman named Betty Dodson, Ph.D., nicknamed the mother of masturbation, called Sex for One: The Joy of Self-Loving that I bought for research purposes for my writing. Possibly we have some other writers out there, if so, you can contact me and hopefully we can correspond about the Zen of Free-Living; Self-Loving; and Self-Healing and Life Learning. I believe you have to think you're important first, in order to heal yourself mentally and physically. I'd like to add the disclaimer that I have no medical degree or psychiatry degree and will not be held legally liable for any statements I impart. You can contact me two ways; I have a blog, Ms. Dodson is now 88-years-old.

www.donsmillerepilepsyexpert.wordpress.com my handle is a joke, a play on the medical: degreelessdrdon, also at strangedetour@grantsburgtelcom.net Feel free to subscribe to my blog and pose questions, if I can't answer them on the spot, I will research them.

Living together/pre-marital sex

Still frowned upon by most churches, though it has become so common today that most couples that come to be married are already living together, and we don't even bother making an issue of it. Clergy, however, could and likely would be de-frocked for immoral behavior.

I'm 53 1/2, single, and haven't had a girlfriend or boyfriend sexually in 24 years, simple mathematics... Two boyfriend/girlfriend split and that makes one and Cherry was into the solo-sex with one of those vibrating plastic bullets. Too much disclosure, I've said before, Cherry Firestone, hot in temperament as hot in sexual desires.

I believe there are five states of sexual being: hetero-sexual; homosexual; bisexual; asexual; and uni-sexual. Opposite sexes; Same sex; both sexes; no sex; and self-sexual.

In regard to asexual, anyone who has grown up with an over-protective mother, smothered by good intentions, kept away from other people, knows what I'm talking about. No socialization with the opposite sex, or the same sex for that matter.

I'm single now but don't find the situation satisfying. I am looking for a companion, other than my service dog, Buddy. If something more develops out of this relationship, it would be a bonus. By the way, the Buddy-dog enjoys hugs and kisses just as much as I do. We've both aged well together, and now share the same hair color. Just as an update, Buddy Miller, 1-01-00 (a New Millennium puppy) to 1-27-14, RIP my good friend, the story of Buddy and my life together is in Milepost 3. Some tell me that a little gray at the temples looks distinguished, and I have to admit, it does look cool. What they don't see is that my hair isn't really strawberry blonde, and it isn't sun-kissed, bleached by the sun. I don't go out in the sun, ever. For one thing, I only burn, for Don S. Miller; it's only three shades of skin: white, pink, red, followed by a blistered, peeling reptilian snake-like skin. My hair is about 80% white, not gray, white...rights now. And with all the crap I've been through in my life I think I've earned every single one. The true reason I don't go out in the sun or if I do it's with a Stetson cowboy hat on is my brain's reaction to excess heat.

Same-sex unions

"The church" is divided on this issue. Many denominations regard such unions as immoral and against the will of God, since he created us male and female. Some denominations and many individuals within the JSACOTMW (myself included) take note that homosexuality seems to be a condition rather than a choice, and would suggest that in the Spirit of the Loving Christ we should give two consenting adults of the same sex who want to commit their lives to each other the same consideration and respect and legal status as two adults of the opposite sex. In the JSACOTMW clergy are prohibited from giving the church's blessing on same-sex unions through any kind of rite. This leaves homosexuals in a bind, because our official position is to condemn (or at least frown upon) sexual intercourse outside of marriage, and yet we refuse to recognize same-sex marriages.

Lesbianism & Homosexuality, Bi-sexuality

See above. The official position of the Jesus Saves All Church of the Muddy Waters is that there is no sin in the condition, but it frowns upon people acting out their sexual preferences by sexual intercourse (or similar sexual relations) outside of marriage.

Heterosexuality

Many Christian traditions affirm heterosexuality as our natural condition, and affirm that God gave to us the gift of our sexuality for the propagation of the human race, and as a way of drawing us together into relationships of love and affection, and as a way of expressing that love and affection.

When you go to a neurologist's appointment they give you two sheets of paper, one is for the physical, one is for the psychiatric. In the psychiatric there is, "Are you capable of reaching pleasure?" Maybe the wording is slightly different. Rate from 1 to 5, 1 being least or none and 5 being damn yes. I always rate my pleasure as being a 5 because I meditate almost daily and have my writing to devote my life to. They are checking for psychiatric side effects. Confusion, stupidity, anger, depression, signs for potential suicidal thoughts and actions. Confusion with my drugs I've had before, not stupidity although some doctors I've seen might differ in their opinion. Anger, no, though I've been on Keppra that can cause Kepprage. I am currently on Fycompa and both those drugs have the potential for extreme agitation (anger). I guess what I'm saying is that you are expected to answer those questions truthfully. Judging your mental health on a pleasure scale, I'm not sure I care for the idea. Self-pleasure, sounds like what we've just been talking about.

ALSO BY DON S. MILLER

Epilepsy Memoir: My 40-Year Detour

Detour: A 40-Year Epilepsy Memoir

Death is Not the End: Unholy Resurrections Volume 1, a novel.

Seizure: Epilepsy Awareness & Epilepsy Education: The 42-Year Formation of One Man's Epilepsy Identity

On 10-31-16 Psychic Gift with a Price: Power of the Icy Flames, Unholy Resurrections Volume 2, and a novel.

& with this one: Epilepsy: The Lightning Storm Within the Brain: My Personal Reflections in Time's Rear-View Mirror

All books are available in RP; LP; and Kindle. Detour... is also available in other e-formats.

ABOUT DON S MILLER:

Growing up, my idol was Superman, that and extreme near-sightedness are the reason I wear these trendy Clark Kent glasses and invisible long underwear 24 hours a day, 7 days a week, 365 days out of the year. That is probably also the reason I named one of my seizure types after him—Superman Seizures, he flies through the air, then lands with a crash like some defective paper airplane.

I was born in 1963, the beginning of the psychedelic sixties, a bit too young to sample any of that free love that was going around. I grew up a Shelby Mustang muscle car, and then in 1974 I had a figurative head on crash with the E word, and became a dented, rusty, surface-scratched Plymouth Duster, not too bright in his headlights. Over the years my body and brain have evolved into the driverless Mercedes-Benz F-015 luxury car. I've never had a driver's license my entire life, nor am I what they'd call mechanically inclined. I know where the key goes in, the gas goes in, and where the smoke and noise comes out. But somehow I'm going to get a Mercedes-Benz F-015, in the future, when I have my driver's license; that is going to happen, it's just a matter of time. I wonder if the bank would be willing to make a loan to an aspiring writer?

I felt it important to relate the body to something we all know a little about, a car; I also felt it important to relate the brain to something we all know a little about, the engine. I was diagnosed with epilepsy in 1974 and have lived with it for 40 years so I know quite a bit about the seizure condition.

Facebook—

https://www.facebook.com/donsmiller1963

https://www.facebook.com/unholyresurrectionsseries

Epilepsy Foundation—

http://epilepsyfoundation.ning.com/profile/DSMiller

On 2-28-2016 the Epilepsy Foundation site went stagnant and shut down. It was there that I met the three E women who were to be beta readers and go through it for errors. I wanted feedback from actual people that had epilepsy. They needn't have bothered as the proofreader for the manuscript not only had a master in theology but a minor in English. I wanted real E people to read it to give the manuscript authenticity. One of the women had a negative reaction to some writing I shared with her though for the life of me I don't know why because she never told. Another woman also had a negative reaction to some of my fiction but didn't say why. I respect them as fellow human beings even though they never respected my writing. They shared other aspects of their psyche that I keep in confidence and will never share. Possibly one of the women will read this book although I have my doubts on that.

Send me a friend request and I won't refuse it.

Email—strangedetour@grantsburgtelcom.net (because in 1974, my life did indeed take a strange detour down an uncharted road)

Google+

http://google.com/+DonMiller1963

Linked In: I have another Linked In page but I'm dipped in pig snort if I can remember it.

http://www.linkedin.com/pub/don-miller/

Twitter:

http://twitter.com/donmillerwrites

http://twitter.com/DonMillerbooks

At the time I add this, @donmillerwrites has 1100 follow-ers, tweet me! Twitter has put a lock on me following any more people, they do that when you reach 2000 but as soon as they let me I'll follow you back. They use some magical formula—the more people follow you, the more you can fol-low; to put that in perspective some people follow tens of thousands people; my old friend Stephen E. King, last time I checked was following 39 people, I've tweeted him but no response unlike author—Barry Eisler, he responds with a personal tweet, good luck on your writing future Barry. I've tried educating people about E on Twitter but it is hard to know if all that medical mud is sticking to anything. It is also hard to tell anything on Twitter at 140 character tweets. On Face-Book I have managed to educate people about E; one woman and former neighbor in Hammond wanted to know about auras; one man wanted to know about root causes—sometimes seizures are idiopathic, meaning they just don't know why you seize, you just do; my seizures are idiopathic, they don't know why I have abnormal brainwaves, they just are.

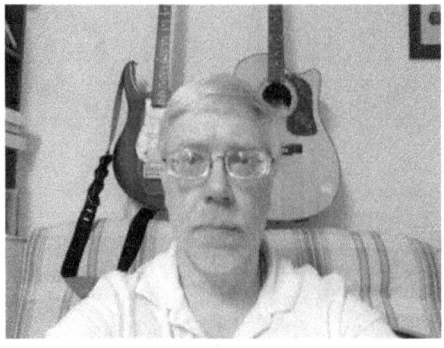

Don S Miller

www.ingramcontent.com/pod-product-compliance
Lightning Source LLC
Chambersburg PA
CBHW080804180526
45168CB00006B/2326